Study of Centenarians

Common Genetic Traits in Those Who Live Past 100

A very short introduction from
The HealthSpan Institute

Study of Centenarians:
Common Genetic Traits in Those Who Live Past 100
A Very Short Introduction from The HealthSpan Institute

ISBN: 9798865593911

Printed in the United States of America

Contents

Chapter 1:
Introduction

Definition of Centenarians.. 13

The Increasing Relevance of Centenarian Studies............. 14

1. Demographic Shifts..15

2. Advances in Medical Research 15

3. Societal Implications of Extended Lifespans...................15

4. Quality of Life Considerations 15

5. Cultural and Psychosocial Insights 16

Objective and Scope of the Book 16

Objective 16

Scope 17

Chapter 2:
The History and Demography of Centenarians

Historical Prevalence of Centenarians 19

Ancient Times 19

Middle Ages to Renaissance 19

18th and 19th Centuries 20

20th Century Onward 20

Today 20

Current Demographic Statistics 21

Global Prevalence 21

Regional Distribution 21

Gender Distribution 22

Urban vs. Rural Distribution...22

Socio-economic Factors..22

Geographic Hotspots and "Blue Zones" 23

Identified Blue Zones 23

Commonalities Among Blue Zones 24

Conclusion 25

Chapter 3:
Basics of Genetics Relevant to Longevity

Overview of human genetics 26

Structure of DNA 26

Genes and Proteins 26

Human Genome 27

Variations and Mutations 27

Inheritance Patterns 27

Genetics and Longevity 28

How Genetics Determine Life Expectancy 28

The Genetic Component of Longevity 28

Key Genes Associated with Longevity 28

Telomeres and Aging 29

Genetic Mutations and Longevity 29

Epigenetics and Aging 29

The Interplay with Environment and Lifestyle 29

Conclusion 30

Common Misconceptions about Genetics and Aging 30

Misconception 1: Aging is Entirely Genetic 30

Misconception 2: There's a Single "Aging Gene" 30

Misconception 3: If My Parents Lived Long Lives, I Will Too 31

Misconception 4: Telomere Length is the Sole
Determinant of Aging 31

Misconception 5: We Can Accurately Predict Our
Lifespan Using Genetics Alone 31

Misconception 6: Genetic Interventions Can
Significantly Extend Human Life.. 31

Misconception 7: Aging is an Unavoidable Decline 32

Chapter 4:
Common Genetic Traits in Centenarians

FOXO3A Gene and Its Significance 33

What is the FOXO3A Gene? 33

Association with Longevity 33

Biological Mechanisms Underlying Its Role 33

Environmental Interactions and FOXO3A 34

FOXO3A in Disease Resistance 34

Conclusion 34

Other Significant Genes and Their Functions 35

APOE Gene 35

SIRT1 Gene 35

IL-6 Gene 36

IGF-1R Gene 36

MTHFR Gene 36

Conclusion 36

Interplay of Genes Leading to Longevity 37

Synergistic Actions 37

Compensatory Mechanisms 37

Epistasis and Gene-Gene Interactions 38

Pathway Convergence 38

Modulation by Environmental Factors 38

Polygenic Nature of Longevity 38

Conclusion 38

Chapter 5:
The Role of Epigenetics in Longevity

Definition and Overview of Epigenetics 40

What is Epigenetics? 40

Key Epigenetic Mechanisms 40

Environmental Influences on Epigenetics.........................41

Epigenetic Memory 41

Epigenetics in Aging and Longevity 41

Conclusion 42

How Epigenetic Changes Affect Aging 42

The Epigenetic Clock 42

Epigenetic Drift and Deregulation 42

Role of Histone Modifications 43

Influence of Non-coding RNAs 43

Environment, Lifestyle, and Epigenetic Aging 43

Conclusion 44

Epigenetic Commonalities Among Centenarians 44

Distinctive DNA Methylation Patterns 44

Conserved Epigenetic Age 45

Histone Modification Profiles 45

Non-coding RNA Expression 45

Response to Environmental Stimuli 45

Stability Amidst Drift..45

Conclusion..46

Chapter 6:
Comparative Analysis

**Genes Common Among Centenarians vs.
General Population 47**

FOXO3A: The Longevity Gene...47

APOE and Cardiovascular Health 47

IGF-1R and Growth Regulation 48

Cholesterol and CETP 48

Telomere Maintenance 48

Other Notable Genes..48

Epigenetic Influences 48

Conclusion 49

The Significance of Telomeres and Telomerase Activity.... 49

Telomeres: Chromosome Protectors 49

Telomerase: The Enzyme of Renewal 50

Centenarians and Telomere Dynamics 50

Telomerase Activity: A Double-Edged Sword................ 50

Telomeres, Telomerase, and Lifestyle............................. 51

Conclusion 51

Other Genetic Variations and Their Implications.............. 51

MTOR Pathway and Cellular Growth 51

SIRTUINS: Guardians of the Genome 52

Klotho: The Anti-Aging Protein 52

HSP70: Cellular Stress Response 52

Angiotensin-Converting Enzyme (ACE) Gene 52

Interactions and Epistasis.. 52

Environmental and Lifestyle Modulators 53

Conclusion 53

Chapter 7:
The Interplay of Genetics and Environment

How External Factors Affect Genetic Expressions 54

Epigenetics: The Bridge Between Genes and Environment........ 54

Nutrition and Dietary Patterns 54

Environmental Toxins and Pollutants 55

Psychological Stress and Trauma 55

Physical Activity 55

Microbial Interactions 55

Circadian Rhythms... 56

Conclusion 56

The Importance of Diet, Exercise, and Stress in Longevity 56

Diet: More Than Just Fuel 56

Exercise: Beyond Physical Fitness 57

Stress: The Silent Accelerator of Aging 58

Conclusion 58

Lifestyle Habits of Centenarians 58

Diverse Diets, Common Themes 59

Consistent Physical Activity 59

Strong Social Ties 59

Stress Management and Mental Resilience 60

Moderation in Vices 60

Conclusion 60

Chapter 8:
Future Directions and Implications

Potential for Genetic Engineering for Longevity 61

Understanding the Genetic Blueprint 61

Current Genetic Engineering Tools 61

Applications and Implications 62

The Road Ahead 63

Conclusion 63

Ethical Considerations 63

Playing God or Advancing Science? 63

Accessibility and Inequality 64

Unintended Consequences 64

Population and Environmental Concerns 64

Cultural and Societal Changes 65

Informed Consent 65

Conclusion 65

The Possibility of Enhancing Human Lifespan Using Findings from Centenarian Studies 66

Translating Genetic Insights 66

Harnessing Epigenetic Knowledge 66

Lifestyle Interventions 67

Challenges and Limitations 67

Broader Implications 67

Conclusion 68

Chapter 9:
Case Studies

Interviews with Centenarians and Their Life Stories 69

Eleanor, 102–New York, USA 69

Hiroshi, 104–Okinawa, Japan 69

Asha, 101–Kerala, India 70

Carlos, 103–Lima, Peru 70

Nadia, 100–Casablanca, Morocco 70

Conclusion 71

Genetic Analysis and Findings 71

Shared Genetic Markers 71

Individual Variations 72

Intriguing Anomalies 72

Shared Epigenetic Changes 72

Conclusion 73

Insights and Lessons from Individual Stories 73

The Importance of Adaptability 73

The Power of Social Connections 74

Living with Purpose 74

The Healing Power of Nature 75

A Balanced Life 75

Conclusion 75

Chapter 10:
Conclusions

Summary of Key Findings 76

   1. Genetic Factors Play a Role 76

   2. Epigenetics Holds Clues 76

   3. The Power of Environment and Lifestyle 77

   4. Blue Zones and Geographic Pockets 77

   5. The Intriguing Anomalies 77

   6. Telomeres and Cellular Aging 77

   7. Personal Narratives are a Treasure Trove 78

   Conclusion 78

The Broader Impact of Understanding the Genetics of Longevity 78

   1. Advancements in Personalized Medicine 78

   2. Prevention Over Cure 79

   3. Economic and Social Implications 79

   4. Environmental Concerns 79

   5. Psychological and Cultural Dimensions 79

   6. Ethical Dilemmas 80

   7. Reimagining Life's Milestones 80

   Conclusion 80

Call to Action for Further Research and Societal Implications 80

   1. Accelerate Multidisciplinary Research 81

   2. Democratisation of Longevity Science 81

   3. Engage with Ethical Debates 81

   4. Public Policy Revisions 81

   5. Education and Outreach 82

   6. Environmental Considerations 82

   7. Document and Celebrate Human Narratives 82

Conclusion 82

Appendix A:
Glossary of Terms

Allele 84

Autosome 84

Centenarian 84

DNA (Deoxyribonucleic Acid) 84

Epigenetics 84

Gene 84

Genome 85

Genotype 85

Gerontology 85

Heterozygous 85

Homozygous 85

Methylation 85

Mitochondria 85

Mutation 85

Phenotype 86

Polymorphism 86

Recessive Gene 86

Telomeres 86

Telomerase 86

Transcription 86

Translation 86

Appendix B:
Detailed Genetic Pathways Discussed

IGF-1 Pathway 88

mTOR Pathway 88

SIRT Pathway 88

AMPK Pathway 89

NRF2 Pathway 89

FOXO Pathways 89

Autophagy Pathway 89

Appendix C:
Resources for Further Reading and Research

Resources for Further Reading and Research 91

Books 91

Journals 92

Online Platforms 92

Organizations and Institutes 93

Chapter 1: Introduction

Definition of Centenarians

A **centenarian** is a person who has reached the age of 100 years or older. The term is derived from the Latin word *centum*, meaning one hundred, combined with the suffix *-arian*, suggesting a relation or connection. In the context of human lifespan, becoming a centenarian is a remarkable feat, often associated with a combination of good genetics, a healthy lifestyle, and favorable environmental factors.

Historically, living to 100 was a rare occurrence. In ancient times, due to factors like disease, lack of medical knowledge, and harsh living conditions, the average human lifespan was much shorter. To become a centenarian in such eras was an exceptional outlier, often attributed to divine favor or extraordinary constitution. However, with the advent of modern medicine, improved living conditions, and a better understanding of health and wellness, the number of centenarians has seen a significant increase in recent decades.

Different cultures and societies have varying ways of recognizing and honoring their centenarians. In many cultures, reaching the age of 100 is celebrated with grand ceremonies and is often accompanied by national or regional recognition. For instance, in the United Kingdom, centenarians receive a birthday card from the reigning monarch. Similarly, in Japan, a country known for its high number of centenarians, there's a national Respect for the Aged Day, where the elderly, especially centenarians, are celebrated and honored.

From a scientific and research perspective, centenarians are of particular interest. They represent a unique demographic that has managed to outlive the average human lifespan by a significant margin. Researchers and scientists study this group to understand the factors contributing to their longevity. The goal is often to decipher the secrets of their extended lifespan and see how these lessons can be applied to the broader population. Their longevity is not just seen as a function of their genetic makeup but also as a result of their lifestyle choices, mental health, community involvement, and other factors that might contribute to prolonged life.

Moreover, it's important to note the distinction between centenarians and supercentenarians. While centenarians have lived for at least 100 years, supercentenarians are those rare individuals who have reached the age of 110 or more. The latter group is even more exclusive and provides an even deeper pool of insights into the extremes of human longevity.

In studying centenarians, there's also a focus on their quality of life. It's not just about the number of years lived, but the richness of experiences, the state of physical and mental health, and the ability to lead a fulfilling life even in the later years. Many centenarians exhibit a zest for life, remain curious, and maintain strong social connections, factors that researchers believe play a crucial role in their extended lifespans.

In conclusion, centenarians are not just individuals who have lived for a century or more; they are emblematic of the pinnacle of human longevity. They serve as inspiring figures, reminding us of the potential for long, fulfilling lives. Through a combination of genetic factors, lifestyle choices, and perhaps a touch of luck, these individuals have surpassed a significant milestone in the human lifespan. By studying them, we hope to unlock the secrets of longevity, paving the way for future generations to lead longer, healthier lives.

The Increasing Relevance of Centenarian Studies

As the global population ages and life expectancy rises, understanding the determinants of healthy aging and longevity becomes increasingly crucial. The study of centenarians—individuals who have reached or surpassed the age of 100—has taken on heightened significance in recent years. This rising relevance can be attributed to several factors, including demographic shifts, advances in medical research, and societal implications of extended lifespans.

1. Demographic Shifts

The 21st century has witnessed significant changes in global demographics. The percentage of the elderly population is steadily increasing in many regions, leading to what many experts term the "aging population" phenomenon. As a result, society grapples with unique challenges, from restructuring healthcare systems to rethinking retirement and labor force dynamics. Understanding the secrets behind the longevity of centenarians can offer valuable insights into addressing these challenges and ensuring that a larger elderly population can lead fulfilling, healthy lives.

2. Advances in Medical Research

Medical science has seen exponential growth over the past few decades. The advances in genomics, biotechnology, and personalized medicine have made it possible to delve deeper into the intricacies of human biology and aging. Centenarians serve as a unique study group in this context. By understanding the genetic, epigenetic, and physiological factors that contribute to their long lives, researchers can potentially identify pathways to enhance healthspan—the period of one's life free from chronic diseases or disability—for the broader population.

3. Societal Implications of Extended Lifespans

The potential to extend human life is both an exciting prospect and a source of ethical, economic, and societal contemplation. If the secrets of centenarians can be unlocked and applied to the broader populace, societies worldwide will have to grapple with implications ranging from overpopulation and resource scarcity to redefining life stages, careers, and family structures. Centenarian studies are thus not just a scientific endeavor but a lens through which to understand and prepare for a rapidly changing societal landscape.

4. Quality of Life Considerations

Living longer is undoubtedly an achievement, but the quality of those extended years is equally important. Centenarians, in many cases, don't just live longer—they often live better, with fewer ailments and a zest for life that defies their age. Studying this demographic can offer insights into cognitive health, mental well-being, and factors that contribute to a rich and fulfilling elderly life. This is particularly relevant as societies aim to shift the focus from mere lifespan to healthspan, emphasizing a life free from debilitating conditions.

5. Cultural and Psychosocial Insights

Beyond the genetic and physiological factors, the study of centenarians provides a treasure trove of cultural and psychosocial insights. From dietary habits to social connections, from mental resilience to cultural practices, understanding the broader environmental and social factors that influence the lives of centenarians can inform public health policies, community programs, and individual lifestyle choices.

In conclusion, the study of centenarians stands at the intersection of science, society, ethics, and culture. As humanity stands on the precipice of potentially transformative discoveries in longevity and health, centenarian studies offer a roadmap, a cautionary tale, and a source of inspiration. Their increasing relevance is a testament to the ever-evolving understanding of life, aging, and the potential of the human body and spirit. As we continue to explore the mysteries of longevity, centenarians will undoubtedly remain at the forefront, guiding our inquiries and shaping our aspirations for a longer, healthier future.

Objective and Scope of the Book

The marvel of human existence is punctuated by the tales of those who have lived a century and beyond, the centenarians. This book's central premise is to delve into the mysteries of longevity, to understand the factors that contribute to an extended lifespan, and to explore what the broader population might learn from the lives of centenarians.

Objective

The primary objective of this book is threefold:

1. **Scientific Exploration**: To provide an overview of the current scientific understanding related to the genetics of centenarians. By shedding light on the genetic commonalities among those who

live past 100, we aim to offer insights into the biological determinants of longevity.

2. **Holistic Understanding**: Beyond genetics, the book aims to explore the lifestyle, environmental, psychological, and societal factors that influence longevity. Recognizing that living a long life isn't solely the result of one's genetic makeup, we delve into the myriad elements that contribute to a life well-lived and extended.

3. **Implications for the Broader Population**: With the insights garnered from studying centenarians, the book seeks to provide recommendations and considerations for the broader population. The goal is to distill lessons that might help others lead not only longer but healthier and more fulfilling lives.

Scope

To achieve these objectives, the book will cover a diverse range of topics and areas of study, including:

Historical and Demographic Overview: Understanding the history of centenarians and examining their demographics across various regions and cultures. This serves as a foundation for subsequent chapters, setting the context for deeper explorations.

Genetic Underpinnings: A look into the genetic traits commonly found among centenarians. This section will delve into specific genes, their functions, and their implications for longevity.

Role of Epigenetics: Exploring how external factors can influence gene expression and its potential impacts on longevity.

Lifestyle and Environmental Factors: Investigating the daily habits, dietary preferences, physical activities, mental health practices, and environmental conditions that are common among centenarians.

Cultural and Societal Perspectives: Examining the societal structures, cultural practices, and community involvement of centenarians across different regions and cultures.

Case Studies: Presenting real-life stories and interviews with centenarians, offering readers a personal glimpse into their lives, challenges, and wisdom.

Future Implications: Discussing the potential of applying findings from centenarian studies to broader public health recommendations, genetic engineering, and ethical considerations.

Although this book is just a short introduction, its scope is broad, aiming to offer readers an understanding of centenarians from various angles. While the scientific aspects form the core of our exploration, the book adopts a multidisciplinary approach, acknowledging that the secret to longevity is multifaceted and influenced by a blend of genetics, environment, society, and personal choices.

In conclusion, this book's ambition is *not* to offer a comprehensive scientific treatise on longevity but to inspire, inform, and provoke thought. Through the lives of centenarians, we find a mirror to our aspirations, fears, and potential. By understanding them, we hope to better understand ourselves and the myriad factors that shape our journey through life. Whether you're a researcher, a student, or simply a curious soul, this book aims to offer insights, lessons, and a deeper appreciation for the marvel of human longevity.

Chapter 2:
The History and Demography of Centenarians

Historical Prevalence of Centenarians

The presence of centenarians, those exceptional individuals who cross the 100-year threshold, has always been a source of fascination, admiration, and intrigue. However, the prevalence of centenarians throughout history has varied greatly, shaped by medical, societal, and environmental contexts of different epochs.

Ancient Times

In ancient civilizations, the average life expectancy was significantly lower than today, often ranging between 20 to 40 years. Factors like infant mortality, lack of medical knowledge, and frequent wars and famines contributed to this lower lifespan. However, textual references from ancient Greece, China, and other cultures do speak of individuals living to advanced ages, though precise ages are often shrouded in myth and exaggeration.

For instance, biblical accounts speak of patriarchs like Methuselah living for hundreds of years, though such accounts are often interpreted symbolically rather than literally. Ancient Chinese texts also mention long-lived sages, suggesting a cultural reverence for longevity.

Middle Ages to Renaissance

The Middle Ages saw slight improvements in life expectancy, particularly with the establishment of more stable societal structures. Still, reaching 100 years remained an exceptional feat. The few centenarians of these eras were often subjects of local folklore, and their longevity was sometimes attributed to divine blessings or unique personal attributes.

During the Renaissance, as records became more systematic and reliable, we see clearer documentation of centenarians. However, even in this era of blossoming knowledge and culture, centenarians remained rare, with the majority of people not living past their 60s.

18th and 19th Centuries

The 18th and 19th centuries marked the beginnings of significant medical and societal advancements. The establishment of public health measures, better sanitation, advancements in medicine, and improvements in nutrition started to have a positive impact on life expectancy. While the average age was on the rise, centenarians, though still rare, began to be recognized and celebrated in more organized ways in various cultures.

20th Century Onward

The 20th century witnessed a seismic shift in the prevalence of centenarians. With rapid advancements in medical science, the discovery of antibiotics, the eradication or control of numerous diseases, and improvements in public health, life expectancy saw dramatic increases. By the latter half of the 20th century, centenarians were no longer extreme rarities but recognized demographics in many countries.

Countries like Japan, with its emphasis on diet, community, and healthcare, began to report significant numbers of centenarians. By the turn of the 21st century, many developed nations had established formal ways to recognize and celebrate their centenarian citizens.

Today

In today's world, the number of centenarians is growing at an unprecedented rate. Predictions suggest that by 2050, there could be over a million centenarians worldwide. This rise is not just due to medical advancements but also increased awareness about healthy lifestyles, mental well-being, and proactive healthcare.

In conclusion, the journey of centenarians through history is a testament to humanity's resilience, adaptability, and progress. From being subjects of myth and reverence in ancient times to becoming focal points of scientific study today, centenarians encapsulate our ever-evolving understanding of life and longevity. Their increasing prevalence in modern times is not just a demographic statistic but a symbol of human achievement and potential.

Current Demographic Statistics

The 21st century, often termed the 'age of longevity', has seen a notable increase in the number of centenarians worldwide. This rise is attributed to a combination of advances in healthcare, improved living conditions, and heightened awareness of healthy lifestyles. Below, we delve into the current demographic statistics of centenarians, offering a snapshot of this remarkable group's global distribution and characteristics.

Global Prevalence

As of recent data leading up to 2022, estimates suggest that there are more than half a million centenarians globally. This number has seen a consistent upward trend over the past few decades, and projections indicate this growth will continue. By 2050, some estimates suggest that the global number of centenarians might surpass one million.

Regional Distribution

Asia: Home to a vast population, Asia has a significant number of centenarians. Japan, in particular, stands out with the highest numbers, especially in regions like Okinawa, often referred to as the "Land of Immortals" due to its high longevity rates.

Europe: Many European countries, especially those in Western Europe, have witnessed a steady rise in their centenarian populations. France, Italy, and Spain are among the countries with notable numbers.

North America: The United States has one of the largest centenarian populations in absolute numbers. Canada, while having fewer centenarians due to its smaller population, showcases similar growth rates in its centenarian demographics.

Oceania: Australia, with its high standard of living and healthcare, has seen consistent growth in its centenarian population over the past few decades.

Africa and South America: While exact numbers are sometimes harder to ascertain due to varying levels of record-keeping, both continents have their share of centenarians. However, the prevalence is generally lower than in some other regions, possibly due to healthcare disparities and other socio-economic factors.

Gender Distribution

One consistent trend globally is the gender disparity among centenarians. Women significantly outnumber men in this age bracket. For instance, in places like Japan and the United States, women constitute around 85-90% of the centenarian population. This disparity can be attributed to a combination of biological, environmental, and lifestyle factors that contribute to the generally higher life expectancy of women.

Urban vs. Rural Distribution

There's a fascinating divide when it comes to the urban and rural distribution of centenarians. While cities offer better healthcare facilities, many 'Blue Zones'—areas in the world known for high longevity rates—are located in more rural or semi-rural settings. These areas, like Okinawa in Japan, Sardinia in Italy, and Nicoya in Costa Rica, often emphasize community living, natural diets, and regular physical activity, all contributing to longer life spans.

Socio-economic Factors

While the data varies across regions, there is often a correlation between socio-economic status and longevity. Access to quality healthcare, nutritious food, education, and a clean environment can significantly influence one's life span. However, it's essential to consider cultural and community factors, as many centenarians from modest backgrounds in 'Blue Zones' lead long, healthy lives due to strong social ties and traditional lifestyles.

In conclusion, the current demographic landscape of centenarians offers a rich tapestry of insights. From the bustling cities of developed nations to the tranquil countryside of 'Blue Zones', centenarians are a testament to the diverse pathways to longevity. As their numbers grow, so does our understanding of life's potential and the myriad factors that shape our journey through the years.

Geographic Hotspots and "Blue Zones"

The global map of longevity is dotted with specific regions known for their unusually high concentrations of centenarians. Often referred to as "Blue Zones", these areas have become focal points of scientific, sociological, and anthropological studies aiming to decode the secrets of longevity. The term "Blue Zone" was popularized by National Geographic explorer and author Dan Buettner, and since its introduction, the concept has captured the world's imagination.

Identified Blue Zones

There are five primary regions that have been distinctly recognized as Blue Zones:

1. **Okinawa, Japan**: Often termed the "Land of Immortals", Okinawa boasts the world's highest prevalence of female centenarians. The Okinawan lifestyle is marked by a plant-heavy diet rich in sweet potatoes, tofu, and vegetables. Their societal structure emphasizes strong community ties, often seen in their local practice called 'moai', a group of close friends who offer social and emotional support throughout life.

2. **Sardinia, Italy**: In the mountainous regions of Sardinia, particularly in the Nuoro province, male centenarians are notably prevalent. A combination of factors, such as a diet rich in whole grains, vegetables, and healthy fats from olive oil and nuts, along with regular physical activity from pastoral and agricultural work, contribute to their longevity.

3. **Nicoya Peninsula, Costa Rica**: The residents of this region benefit from a diet rich in tropical fruits, beans, rice, and corn. Moreover, the 'plan de vida' or 'reason to live' ethos that permeates the Nicoyan culture emphasizes the importance of having a purpose, especially in one's later years.

4. **Ikaria, Greece**: This Aegean island has one of the highest rates of nonagenarians globally. Factors contributing to this include a Mediterranean diet rich in vegetables, legumes, and olive oil, limited processed foods, and an active lifestyle. Additionally, Ikarians maintain robust social connections and frequently partake in community events.

5. **Loma Linda, California**: A bit of an outlier, this region in the U.S. is known for its significant population of Seventh-day Adventists. Their religious beliefs promote a vegetarian diet, regular exercise, and a strong sense of community, all of which are factors believed to contribute to their extended life expectancy.

Commonalities Among Blue Zones

While each Blue Zone has its unique characteristics, several commonalities can be observed across these regions:

Diet: Natural, locally sourced, and plant-heavy diets are a hallmark of Blue Zones. Processed foods are limited, and there's an emphasis on whole foods rich in antioxidants and nutrients.

Physical Activity: Rather than structured exercise routines, residents of Blue Zones engage in natural, daily physical activities like farming, walking, or traditional dances.

Social Connections: Strong social bonds, whether through family, friends, or community, play a crucial role in mental well-being and longevity.

Sense of Purpose: Whether it's through religious beliefs, community roles, or familial responsibilities, having a clear sense of purpose is a common trait among Blue Zone residents.

Moderate Consumption: Whether it's food, alcohol, or other indulgences, moderation is a consistent theme. For instance, the Okinawan principle of 'Hara hachi bu' encourages eating until one is 80% full.

Conclusion

Blue Zones offer a window into lifestyles and cultures that nurture longevity. While genetics undoubtedly play a role, it's evident that environmental, societal, and personal habits significantly impact one's lifespan. As the global community grapples with the challenges of an aging population, the lessons from these geographic hotspots become increasingly relevant, urging us to reevaluate and perhaps realign our modern lifestyles.

Chapter 3: Basics of Genetics Relevant to Longevity

Overview of human genetics

When diving into the study of centenarians and the genetic traits that might predispose individuals to live past 100, it's essential first to have a basic understanding of human genetics. Genetics, at its core, is the study of genes, the hereditary units of life. These genes determine everything from the color of our eyes to our susceptibility to certain diseases.

Structure of DNA

Every cell in our body contains a nucleus, and within this nucleus are chromosomes made up of long strands of DNA (Deoxyribonucleic Acid). DNA consists of two intertwined helices, creating its characteristic double-helix structure. These helices are made up of four chemical units or bases: Adenine (A), Thymine (T), Cytosine (C), and Guanine (G).

These bases pair up in specific ways: A with T and C with G. The sequence in which these bases appear determines the information contained in a segment of DNA.

Genes and Proteins

Segments of DNA that carry the instructions to make a particular protein are known as genes. Proteins are vital for our body's structure and function—everything from building tissues to driving chemical reactions.

When a protein needs to be made, the DNA segment (or gene) specific to that protein is read and transcribed into RNA (Ribonucleic Acid). This RNA is then translated into the protein. Any errors or mutations in the DNA sequence can affect the final protein's structure or function, potentially leading to diseases or unique traits.

Human Genome

The entire set of DNA in our bodies, encompassing around 20,000-25,000 genes, is known as the human genome. In 2003, the Human Genome Project successfully mapped out the entire sequence of the human genome, marking a monumental achievement in the field of genetics.

Variations and Mutations

While all humans share a vast majority of their DNA, it's the small variations that make us unique. These variations can affect everything from our physical appearance to our likelihood of developing certain diseases.

A mutation refers to a change in the DNA sequence. While the term "mutation" might conjure images of harmful changes, many mutations are benign, having no discernible impact on our health or function. Some mutations, however, can confer advantages or lead to genetic disorders.

Inheritance Patterns

Genes are passed down from parents to offspring. Humans have 23 pairs of chromosomes: one pair of sex chromosomes (determining gender) and 22 pairs of autosomes. One chromosome from each pair is inherited from the mother and the other from the father.

There are several patterns of genetic inheritance:

- **Dominant**: Where only one mutated copy of a gene is needed to express a trait or disorder.
- **Recessive**: Where two mutated copies (one from each parent) are needed to express a trait or disorder.
- **X-linked**: Where the gene causing the trait or disorder is located on the X chromosome.

Genetics and Longevity

As we delve deeper into the genetics of longevity, it's crucial to remember that longevity is likely influenced by a combination of multiple genes, environmental factors, and lifestyle choices. While certain genetic markers might predispose individuals to live longer, they are just one piece of the intricate puzzle of human life and aging.

By grounding ourselves in these basics of genetics, we can better appreciate and understand the genetic intricacies that might play a role in the remarkable longevity of centenarians.

How Genetics Determine Life Expectancy

Life expectancy, defined as the average number of years an individual can expect to live, is influenced by a confluence of factors ranging from environmental conditions to lifestyle choices. However, amidst these variables, genetics plays a pivotal role. By understanding how our genes affect longevity, we can glean insights into the biological mechanisms underlying the aging process and, consequently, lifespan.

The Genetic Component of Longevity

It's estimated that about 20-30% of an individual's lifespan can be attributed to genetics, while the remainder is influenced by environmental and lifestyle factors. This estimate arises from studies on familial longevity, especially those focusing on siblings and twins. Identical twins, who share 100% of their genes, often have more similar lifespans compared to fraternal twins or siblings, highlighting the genetic influence.

Key Genes Associated with Longevity

Several genes have been identified as being linked to longevity. Some of the most notable ones include:

- **FOXO3**: Part of the FOXO gene family, FOXO3 has been consistently associated with human longevity across multiple populations. It plays a role in regulating the insulin/IGF-1 signaling pathway, which affects metabolism and cellular growth.

- **APOE**: The apolipoprotein E gene is linked to cholesterol metabolism and has variants associated with either increased risk of Alzheimer's disease or enhanced longevity.
- **SIRT1**: This gene is involved in DNA repair and cellular regulation. It's believed to play a role in delaying the aging process and extending lifespan.

Telomeres and Aging

Telomeres, the protective caps at the ends of our chromosomes, play a crucial role in aging. Each time a cell divides, the telomeres shorten. When they become too short, the cell can no longer divide and becomes inactive or senescent or dies. The length and rate of telomere shortening are believed to be genetically determined, with longer telomeres being associated with longer lifespans and a reduced risk of age-related diseases.

Genetic Mutations and Longevity

Not all genetic influences on lifespan are beneficial. Some genetic mutations can lead to early-onset diseases or conditions that reduce an individual's lifespan. However, understanding these adverse genetic influences can offer insights into the biology of aging and potential interventions.

Epigenetics and Aging

While our DNA sequence plays a role in determining lifespan, how genes are expressed is equally crucial. Epigenetics, which refers to changes in gene expression without alterations to the underlying DNA sequence, has emerged as a key player in aging. Environmental factors, lifestyle choices, and even early-life experiences can lead to epigenetic modifications, influencing the aging process and, consequently, lifespan.

The Interplay with Environment and Lifestyle

While genetics lays the foundation for potential longevity, interactions with environmental and lifestyle factors can either enhance or diminish this potential. For example, an individual with a genetic predisposition for longevity might not achieve that potential if they adopt unhealthy habits or live in an environment with poor healthcare or significant pollution.

Conclusion

The intricate dance between genetics and life expectancy is an ongoing area of research. While we've identified certain genes and genetic processes that influence longevity, the full picture remains complex and multifaceted. However, one thing is clear: while our genes provide a blueprint for potential longevity, the choices we make and the environment we live in play pivotal roles in realizing that potential.

By understanding the genetic basis of longevity, we can develop strategies and interventions to harness our genetic potential, paving the way for longer, healthier lives.

Common Misconceptions about Genetics and Aging

In the world of genetics and aging, misconceptions are rife. These misconceptions stem from a combination of outdated beliefs, oversimplifications in popular media, and misinterpretations of complex scientific data. This section aims to debunk some of the most common misconceptions surrounding genetics and the aging process.

Misconception 1: Aging is Entirely Genetic

Truth: While genetics play a role in determining our lifespan and healthspan, they're only part of the picture. Lifestyle, environment, and random cellular events also contribute significantly. Some studies suggest that genetics may account for only about 25% of the variation in human lifespan. Thus, while inheriting "good genes" can be advantageous, it's no guarantee of reaching centenarian status without the right environmental and lifestyle factors.

Misconception 2: There's a Single "Aging Gene"

Truth: Aging is a complex process influenced by numerous genes, not just one "master switch." While certain genes, like FOXO3A or telomerase, have a more pronounced effect on lifespan, no single gene controls the entire aging process. Instead, a network of genes interacts with environmental factors to determine how quickly we age and how susceptible we are to age-related diseases.

Misconception 3: If My Parents Lived Long Lives, I Will Too

Truth: While having long-lived ancestors can increase your chances of living a longer life, it doesn't guarantee it. As mentioned, environmental and lifestyle factors play a massive role. For instance, a person with long-lived genes who smokes, eats poorly, and avoids exercise might not live as long as their genes might predict.

Misconception 4: Telomere Length is the Sole Determinant of Aging

Truth: Telomeres, the protective caps at the ends of our chromosomes, do play a role in aging. Shortened telomeres are associated with increased disease risk and earlier death. However, telomere length is just one piece of the longevity puzzle. Many other factors, both genetic and environmental, contribute to the aging process.

Misconception 5: We Can Accurately Predict Our Lifespan Using Genetics Alone

Truth: Despite advances in genetic research, predicting an individual's lifespan remains challenging. While certain genetic markers can indicate predispositions to particular diseases or health outcomes, many other factors—some genetic, others environmental or random—will influence actual lifespan.

Misconception 6: Genetic Interventions Can Significantly Extend Human Life

Truth: While certain genetic interventions have shown promise in extending the lives of model organisms like worms, flies, and mice, translating these findings to humans is not straightforward. Humans have longer lifespans and more genetic complexity than these organisms, making the effects of interventions less predictable. While there's potential in genetic research to improve healthspan (the period of life spent in good health), it's uncertain how much human lifespan can be extended through genetic means alone.

Misconception 7: Aging is an Unavoidable Decline

Truth: Aging is not synonymous with inevitable decline. Many physiological changes with age are adaptive, not degenerative. For instance, certain cognitive abilities, like wisdom and problem-solving, can improve with age. Understanding the distinction between pathological aging (disease-driven) and "normal" or healthy aging is crucial.

In conclusion, while genetics provide a window into the intricacies of aging, they are just one piece of a much larger puzzle. As research continues to evolve, it's crucial to approach the topic with nuance, recognizing the interplay between our genes, our choices, and our environment. Dispelling these misconceptions allows for a more informed and proactive approach to our own aging processes.

Chapter 4:
Common Genetic Traits in Centenarians

FOXO3A Gene and Its Significance

The study of genetics in the context of longevity has brought several genes into the limelight, but few have garnered as much attention and scientific interest as the FOXO3A gene. Predominantly known for its association with increased lifespan across multiple populations, the FOXO3A gene offers insights into the biology of aging and the intricate mechanisms underlying longevity.

What is the FOXO3A Gene?

FOXO3A is a member of the FOXO family of transcription factors, proteins that regulate the expression of target genes. This gene encodes a transcription factor that plays a pivotal role in numerous cellular processes, including metabolism, cell cycle arrest, apoptosis (programmed cell death), DNA repair, and oxidative stress resistance.

Association with Longevity

Several genetic studies have consistently identified variants of the FOXO3A gene to be associated with longevity. In diverse populations, from Americans to Japanese to Europeans, specific alleles (gene variants) of FOXO3A have been found to be more prevalent among centenarians and supercentenarians (those aged over 110 years) than in the general population.

Biological Mechanisms Underlying Its Role

The significance of FOXO3A in longevity can be attributed to multiple pathways it influences:

- **Cellular Stress Resistance**: FOXO3A promotes the expression of genes that combat oxidative stress. By bolstering the cell's defenses against reactive oxygen species, it reduces cellular damage, a key factor in aging.

- **DNA Repair**: FOXO3A upregulates genes involved in DNA repair. Enhanced DNA repair mechanisms can counteract genomic instability, a hallmark of aging.

- **Cell Cycle Regulation**: The protein product of FOXO3A can induce cell cycle arrest, preventing damaged cells from dividing and potentially becoming cancerous.

- **Apoptosis**: FOXO3A can trigger apoptosis in damaged or non-functional cells, ensuring they don't accumulate and cause tissue dysfunction.

- **Metabolism**: FOXO3A influences insulin signaling and glucose metabolism, crucial processes linked to lifespan and age-related diseases like diabetes.

Environmental Interactions and FOXO3A

Interestingly, the activity of the FOXO3A transcription factor is influenced by environmental factors. For instance, dietary restriction, known to extend lifespan in several organisms, enhances the activity of FOXO3A, leading to increased expression of its target genes. Similarly, physical activity has been shown to modulate FOXO3A activity, suggesting a potential link between exercise, this gene, and longevity.

FOXO3A in Disease Resistance

Apart from direct influences on aging, the FOXO3A gene has implications for age-related diseases. Variants of this gene have been linked to reduced risks of certain cancers, cardiovascular diseases, and neurodegenerative conditions. The protective mechanisms are believed to stem from the gene's role in DNA repair, oxidative stress resistance, and metabolic regulation.

Conclusion

The FOXO3A gene stands as a testament to the intricate and multifaceted nature of the genetics of longevity. Its diverse roles, from cellular protection to metabolic regulation, highlight the interconnectedness of biological processes in determining lifespan.

For researchers and scientists aiming to decipher the secrets of centenarians, the FOXO3A gene provides a valuable piece of the puzzle. As we continue to explore its nuances and interactions, it might pave the way for therapeutic strategies aiming to harness its protective effects, potentially extending healthspan and lifespan in the broader population.

Other Significant Genes and Their Functions

While the FOXO3A gene has earned a reputation for its association with longevity, it's just one piece in the intricate genetic tapestry of centenarians. Multiple genes, often interacting in complex ways, contribute to the exceptional lifespan and healthspan of these individuals. Here, we explore some of the other significant genes associated with longevity and their primary functions.

APOE Gene

Function: The APOE gene encodes apolipoprotein E, a protein primarily involved in lipid metabolism and cholesterol transport in the bloodstream.

Significance in Longevity: Certain variants of the APOE gene, especially the ε2 allele, have been linked to increased lifespan. Conversely, the ε4 allele is associated with a higher risk of Alzheimer's disease and cardiovascular diseases. Many centenarians possess the ε2 allele, suggesting its potential protective effects.

SIRT1 Gene

Function: SIRT1 is one of the sirtuins, a family of proteins involved in cellular health and metabolism. SIRT1 plays roles in DNA repair, inflammation reduction, and metabolic regulation.

Significance in Longevity: Activation of SIRT1, akin to FOXO3A, is associated with lifespan extension in various organisms. In humans, certain

SIRT1 variants have been linked to longevity, especially in populations with high numbers of centenarians.

IL-6 Gene

Function: The IL-6 gene encodes interleukin-6, a cytokine (a type of signaling protein) involved in inflammation and immune response.

Significance in Longevity: Chronic inflammation is considered a hallmark of aging. Variants of the IL-6 gene associated with reduced interleukin-6 production have been found more frequently in centenarians, suggesting that lower inflammatory states might contribute to prolonged lifespan.

IGF-1R Gene

Function: IGF-1R encodes the insulin-like growth factor 1 receptor. This receptor plays a crucial role in growth, development, and metabolism.

Significance in Longevity: Variants of the IGF-1R gene have been identified in centenarian populations, suggesting a possible role in longevity. Reduced IGF-1 signaling, similar to reduced insulin signaling, has been linked to lifespan extension in several organisms.

MTHFR Gene

Function: The MTHFR gene encodes methylenetetrahydrofolate reductase, an enzyme involved in processing amino acids and forming folate compounds.

Significance in Longevity: Specific variants of the MTHFR gene have been associated with longevity. These variants may influence homocysteine metabolism, affecting cardiovascular health and potentially contributing to extended lifespan.

Conclusion

The quest to pinpoint the genetic underpinnings of longevity has uncovered a constellation of genes, each influencing different pathways and processes. From metabolism and inflammation to DNA repair and cellular health, these genes shed light on the multifaceted nature of aging and lifespan.

It's worth noting that genes do not act in isolation. The interplay between these genes, influenced by environmental factors and lifestyle choices, orchestrates the remarkable longevity observed in centenarians. As we continue to map the genetic landscape of those who live past 100, we gain valuable insights that could pave the way for interventions promoting healthy aging for all.

Interplay of Genes Leading to Longevity

Longevity is a complex trait influenced by a symphony of genetic factors, each contributing its unique note. While it's tempting to attribute extended lifespan to individual "longevity genes," it's the intricate interplay of these genes that holds the key to understanding the secrets of centenarians. In this section, we explore how these genes interact, collectively sculpting the genetic blueprint for a prolonged, healthy life.

Synergistic Actions

Many genes associated with longevity don't operate in isolation. Their effects can be synergistic, meaning the combined impact of two or more genes is greater than the sum of their individual effects. For instance, while FOXO3A might enhance cellular stress resistance and DNA repair, its effects could be amplified when combined with the protective actions of SIRT1, which also promotes cellular health. Such synergistic interactions can lead to a robust defense against age-related deterioration.

Compensatory Mechanisms

Some genetic variants might have detrimental effects, potentially increasing susceptibility to certain diseases or accelerating aging. However, centenarians might possess other protective genetic factors that compensate for these adverse effects. For instance, while an individual might carry the APOE ε4 allele, increasing the risk of Alzheimer's, the presence of a beneficial FOXO3A variant might counteract this risk, fostering cognitive health into advanced age.

Epistasis and Gene-Gene Interactions

Epistasis refers to the phenomenon where the effect of one gene is modified by one or several other genes. In the context of longevity, this means that the influence of a particular gene on lifespan might be dependent on the presence or absence of other genes. Understanding these intricate gene-gene interactions is crucial to demystifying the genetic architecture of longevity.

Pathway Convergence

Many longevity genes converge on common cellular pathways. For instance, both FOXO3A and SIRT1 influence the insulin/IGF-1 signaling pathway, known to affect lifespan in multiple organisms. By targeting the same pathways, multiple genes can collectively modulate cellular processes, enhancing resilience against age-related challenges.

Modulation by Environmental Factors

The expression and activity of longevity genes can be influenced by environmental and lifestyle factors. For example, dietary restriction, known to extend lifespan, can modulate the activity of multiple genes, including those in the FOXO and sirtuin families. Such external factors can influence the interplay of longevity genes, either enhancing or diminishing their effects.

Polygenic Nature of Longevity

Recent studies suggest that longevity is a polygenic trait, meaning it's influenced by many genes, each contributing a small effect. Rather than a few "magic bullet" genes, it's the cumulative effect of numerous beneficial genetic variants that paves the way for a prolonged lifespan. This polygenic landscape underscores the importance of understanding gene-gene interactions and the collective impact of multiple genetic factors.

Conclusion

The interplay of genes leading to longevity is a testament to the complexity and elegance of human biology. It's not just the presence of specific genes but how they interact, compensate for each other, and converge on common pathways that determines one's genetic predisposition to a long, healthy life.

For scientists and researchers, deciphering this intricate web of interactions is both a challenge and an opportunity. As we untangle the genetic symphony of centenarians, we inch closer to potential interventions that harness these insights, promoting health and vitality across the lifespan.

Chapter 5: The Role of Epigenetics in Longevity

Definition and Overview of Epigenetics

In the quest to understand the intricacies of human biology, genetics offers a foundational blueprint. However, if our DNA is the script, epigenetics is the director, subtly influencing how that script is expressed. Delving into the realm of epigenetics uncovers layers of regulation that play pivotal roles in health, disease, and, as emerging evidence suggests, longevity.

What is Epigenetics?

Epigenetics refers to modifications on or around the DNA molecule that don't change the underlying DNA sequence but influence gene activity. These modifications act as molecular switches, turning genes on or off, or modulating their activity levels. In essence, while our DNA provides the information, epigenetic changes dictate how that information is interpreted and acted upon by the cell.

Key Epigenetic Mechanisms

The world of epigenetics is vast, but a few core mechanisms stand out:

- **DNA Methylation:** This involves the addition of a methyl group to a cytosine base in the DNA. Methylation generally represses gene activity, preventing transcription, the first step in gene expression.

- **Histone Modifications:** Histones are proteins around which DNA winds. Modifications to these proteins, such as acetylation or methylation, can influence gene expression by altering the structure of the chromatin (the combination of DNA and proteins).

- **Non-coding RNAs:** These are RNA molecules that don't code for proteins but can influence gene expression and activity. Examples include microRNAs (miRNAs) and long non-coding RNAs (lncRNAs).

Environmental Influences on Epigenetics

One of the fascinating aspects of epigenetics is its dynamic nature. While our DNA sequence remains largely static throughout life, epigenetic marks can change in response to environmental factors. Diet, stress, exposure to toxins, physical activity, and even experiences in early life can induce epigenetic modifications, influencing health and disease trajectories.

Epigenetic Memory

A unique aspect of epigenetics is its potential to confer a form of cellular memory. Certain epigenetic marks can be inherited when a cell divides, ensuring the daughter cells "remember" their identity and function. In some instances, epigenetic changes can even be passed from one generation to the next, although the mechanisms and implications of such transgenerational epigenetic inheritance remain areas of active research.

Epigenetics in Aging and Longevity

Aging is accompanied by a host of epigenetic alterations. Some of these changes may be a result of accumulated environmental exposures over time, while others might be programmed responses. Researchers have identified specific epigenetic patterns, often termed the "epigenetic clock," which correlate with chronological age and can predict biological age with remarkable accuracy.

Interestingly, deviations between this epigenetic clock and chronological age might offer insights into an individual's health and longevity. For instance, an "older" epigenetic age compared to one's actual age might signal increased health risks.

Conclusion

Epigenetics bridges the gap between our genetic code and the myriad environmental factors we encounter throughout life. By offering a mechanism through which external influences can shape gene expression, epigenetics provides a deeper understanding of health, disease, and the biology of aging.

As research in this realm expands, particularly in the context of longevity, epigenetics promises to unveil strategies and interventions that can modulate the aging process, potentially extending not just lifespan, but healthspan as well.

How Epigenetic Changes Affect Aging

The relationship between aging and epigenetics is like the intricate dance of two partners, each influencing the other's movements. As we age, our epigenetic landscape shifts, and these changes, in turn, influence the aging process itself. Understanding the dynamics of this relationship offers a fresh perspective on aging, potentially unveiling strategies to slow its progression and enhance healthspan.

The Epigenetic Clock

One of the most groundbreaking discoveries in the realm of aging and epigenetics is the concept of the "epigenetic clock." By examining patterns of DNA methylation across various sites in the genome, researchers have devised algorithms that can predict an individual's chronological age with startling accuracy. More intriguingly, deviations between the predicted "biological" age and actual age can provide insights into an individual's health and longevity.

For instance, if one's epigenetic age is faster than their chronological age, it might indicate accelerated biological aging and associated health risks. Conversely, a slower epigenetic age might suggest a more youthful biology.

Epigenetic Drift and Deregulation

As we age, our epigenetic marks can become less precise, leading to what's termed "epigenetic drift." This drift might result in genes that should be silent becoming active or active genes becoming repressed. Such deregulation can disturb cellular functions and contribute to aging phenotypes and age-related diseases.

Role of Histone Modifications

Histones, the proteins around which DNA winds, undergo various modifications that influence chromatin structure and gene expression. Aging has been associated with changes in histone modifications, impacting the accessibility of genes. Alterations in histone acetylation and methylation patterns can lead to aberrant gene expression, potentially contributing to cellular senescence, a state of irreversible cell cycle arrest associated with aging.

Influence of Non-coding RNAs

Aging also influences the expression of non-coding RNAs, particularly microRNAs (miRNAs). These small molecules can bind to messenger RNAs (mRNAs), preventing their translation into proteins. Changes in miRNA expression profiles with age can influence various cellular processes, from inflammation and metabolism to DNA repair and cellular stress responses.

Environment, Lifestyle, and Epigenetic Aging

Environmental and lifestyle factors play a significant role in shaping our epigenetic landscape. Factors like dietary patterns, physical activity, stress, and toxin exposure can induce epigenetic changes, influencing aging trajectories. For instance:

- **Diet**: Nutrients can act as epigenetic modulators. Diets rich in methyl donors, such as folate, can influence DNA methylation patterns. Additionally, caloric restriction, known to extend lifespan in various organisms, induces a myriad of epigenetic changes that promote cellular health and resilience.

- **Physical Activity**: Exercise induces changes in DNA methylation and histone modifications, influencing genes related to muscle growth, metabolism, and inflammation.

- **Stress**: Chronic stress can alter epigenetic marks, especially in genes related to the stress response, potentially accelerating aging processes.

Conclusion

Aging and epigenetics are deeply intertwined, with changes in the epigenome influencing the aging process and vice versa. By mapping these changes and understanding their implications, researchers hope to uncover strategies to modulate epigenetic marks, thereby influencing the aging trajectory.

As we continue to unravel the complexities of the epigenome and its role in aging, there's a growing hope that epigenetics might offer a frontier for interventions that enhance healthspan, ensuring not just longer lives, but healthier, more vibrant ones.

Epigenetic Commonalities Among Centenarians

When investigating the secrets to reaching the age of 100 and beyond, genetics offers part of the story. Yet, equally compelling are the epigenetic signatures centenarians share, potentially illuminating how they elude many age-related diseases and maintain robust health. This section delves into the unique epigenetic landscape of centenarians, offering insights into the nexus of epigenetics and exceptional longevity.

Distinctive DNA Methylation Patterns

One of the most striking findings in the study of centenarian epigenetics is the distinctive patterns of DNA methylation they exhibit. While some age-associated methylation patterns are universal, centenarians often display unique marks not commonly found in the average aging population.

In particular, certain genes linked to longevity and age-related diseases, such as those involved in inflammation, DNA repair, and metabolic processes, seem to have differential methylation patterns in centenarians. These patterns might modulate the activity of these genes, conferring protective benefits against age-associated decline.

Conserved Epigenetic Age

Interestingly, while centenarians have surpassed a century of life, their epigenetic clocks often indicate a younger biological age. In essence, while they are chronologically older, their epigenetic age tends to be decelerated. This discrepancy suggests that centenarians may experience slower biological aging, which could be a factor in their extended healthspan and lifespan.

Histone Modification Profiles

Studies indicate that centenarians possess unique histone modification patterns. For instance, certain histone marks associated with active gene expression are enriched in centenarians, especially in genes related to cellular stress responses and DNA repair. Such modifications could contribute to enhanced cellular resilience, allowing centenarians to better counteract age-related challenges.

Non-coding RNA Expression

Centenarians also exhibit distinct profiles of non-coding RNAs, particularly microRNAs (miRNAs). Some miRNAs upregulated in centenarians are known to target pathways associated with inflammation, cellular senescence, and apoptosis. The unique miRNA landscape of centenarians might fine-tune the expression of genes pivotal to longevity, thereby offering a protective edge.

Response to Environmental Stimuli

While the genetic component of longevity is significant, centenarians' interactions with their environment, coupled with their epigenetic responses, are also crucial. Factors like diet, physical activity, and psychosocial well-being might induce favorable epigenetic modifications in centenarians. For example, diets rich in polyphenols, common in regions known for longevity, can influence DNA methylation and histone modification patterns, promoting cellular health.

Stability Amidst Drift

A paradoxical finding in centenarian epigenetics is the combination of stability and flexibility. While certain epigenetic marks seem preserved, offering stability, there's also an adaptive component. Centenarians appear adept at modulating their epigenetic responses to changing environments, ensuring cellular functions are maintained optimally.

Conclusion

The epigenetic tapestry of centenarians is a testament to the intricate interplay of genes, environment, and time. While certain genetic factors undoubtedly predispose individuals to extended lifespans, it's the epigenetic orchestration of these genes, sculpted by life experiences and environmental interactions, that truly shines a light on the secrets of centenarians.

As we further decode the epigenetic commonalities among the world's oldest individuals, we move closer to understanding the symphony of factors that contribute to exceptional longevity, potentially unlocking interventions that can extend healthspan for the wider population.

Chapter 6: Comparative Analysis

Genes Common Among Centenarians vs. General Population

The age-old quest to uncover the secrets of longevity has been re-juvenated with modern genetic research. An interesting approach is to compare the genetic make-up of centenarians—those who have crossed the 100-year threshold—with that of the general population. What makes centenarians unique? And can their genetic makeup provide insights into the pathways and mechanisms underpinning their extended lifespans?

FOXO3A: The Longevity Gene

As previously discussed in Chapter IV, the FOXO3A gene stands out as a significant contributor to the longevity phenotype. It plays a pivotal role in stress resistance, metabolism, and cellular maintenance. While variations of this gene are present in the general population, certain polymorphisms appear at a higher frequency among centenarians, suggesting a potential protective effect against age-related decline.

APOE and Cardiovascular Health

The APOE gene, associated with cholesterol transport and cardiovascular health, presents differently in centenarians versus the general populace. The APOE ε4 allele, linked with a higher risk of Alzheimer's disease and cardiovascular problems, is found at a lower frequency in centenarians. On the contrary, the APOE ε2 allele, believed to be protective against Alzheimer's and cardiovascular diseases, is more common among the exceptionally old.

IGF-1R and Growth Regulation

The Insulin-like Growth Factor 1 Receptor (IGF-1R) plays a role in growth and development. Mutations in the IGF-1R gene, which can affect body size and metabolism, appear more frequently in centenarians. These mutations might modulate the IGF-1 pathway, impacting longevity by altering growth, cellular repair, and metabolic functions.

Cholesterol and CETP

The Cholesteryl Ester Transfer Protein (CETP) gene is another point of difference. Certain variants of the CETP gene are associated with increased HDL cholesterol (often dubbed "good cholesterol") levels and larger HDL particle size. These beneficial cholesterol profiles, more common in centenarians, might offer protection against cardiovascular diseases.

Telomere Maintenance

Telomeres, the protective caps at the ends of chromosomes, shorten as cells divide. Shorter telomeres are associated with aging and a higher risk of age-related diseases. Certain genetic variations linked to telomere length have been identified in centenarians, suggesting that genes involved in telomere maintenance could contribute to their longevity.

Other Notable Genes

In addition to the aforementioned genes, many others show varying frequencies between centenarians and the broader population. These include genes associated with inflammation, DNA repair, cellular senescence, and autophagy. The cumulative effect of these genes might create a biological environment conducive to longevity.

Epigenetic Influences

While genetic predispositions are significant, they aren't the sole determinants of longevity. As explored in earlier chapters, epigenetic modifications can modulate gene expression, potentially enhancing longevity pathways even in the absence of specific genetic variations.

Conclusion

Comparing the genetic landscape of centenarians with the general population offers a unique window into the biology of aging. The increased or decreased frequencies of certain genes and their variants among centenarians hint at the genetic orchestration underpinning extended health and life.

While the genetics of longevity is complex, encompassing myriad genes and pathways, understanding these differences can offer clues to interventions, lifestyle adjustments, and potential therapies that might enhance healthspan and, perhaps, lifespan in the broader population.

The Significance of Telomeres and Telomerase Activity

Telomeres and telomerase activity stand as cornerstones in the study of aging and longevity. These genetic features play crucial roles in cellular aging, health, and overall lifespan. By comparing telomere length and telomerase activity among centenarians and the general population, we can glean vital insights into their contribution to exceptional longevity.

Telomeres: Chromosome Protectors

Telomeres are repetitive DNA sequences found at the ends of chromosomes. Often likened to the plastic tips on shoelaces, they protect chromosomes from deterioration or from fusing with neighboring chromosomes. As cells divide, telomeres shorten—a process associated with aging, cellular dysfunction, and eventual cellular senescence or apoptosis.

Shortened telomeres are not just markers of aging; they also contribute to the aging process itself. Critically short telomeres can cause DNA damage responses, leading to cellular malfunction or enhanced susceptibility to diseases like cancer.

Telomerase: The Enzyme of Renewal

While the natural course involves telomere shortening over time, there's a counteracting force: the enzyme telomerase. Telomerase can add DNA sequences to the ends of chromosomes, thereby extending telomere length and potentially delaying the aging process of the cell. However, in most adult somatic cells, telomerase activity is low or absent, leading to progressive telomere shortening with each cell division.

Interestingly, high telomerase activity is observed in stem cells, germline cells, and many cancer cells. In these cells, telomerase helps maintain telomere length, promoting cellular renewal or unchecked growth, as seen in cancers.

Centenarians and Telomere Dynamics

Studies have shown that centenarians, and often their offspring, possess longer telomeres compared to age-matched controls from the general population. This longer telomere length might contribute to the extended healthspan and lifespan observed in these individuals.

Furthermore, some evidence suggests that centenarians might maintain telomere length better over time. This superior maintenance could stem from genetic predispositions, healthier lifestyles, or a combination of factors that minimize telomere erosion.

Telomerase Activity: A Double-Edged Sword

Elevated telomerase activity can indeed promote telomere elongation and delay cellular aging. Yet, it's a complex balance. As mentioned, many cancer cells upregulate telomerase, enabling these cells to divide uncontrollably. Thus, while augmenting telomerase activity might seem an attractive route for promoting longevity, it could also increase cancer risks.

Interestingly, studies on centenarians hint at a balanced regulation of telomerase activity, where it's sufficiently active to support cellular health but not overly active to predispose to malignancies.

Telomeres, Telomerase, and Lifestyle

It's worth noting that genetics isn't the sole determinant of telomere length and function. Lifestyle factors, including diet, exercise, stress, and sleep, can influence telomere dynamics. Chronic stress, for instance, has been linked to accelerated telomere shortening. Conversely, certain interventions, like meditation and regular exercise, might help preserve telomere length.

Conclusion

In the realm of comparative analysis, telomeres and telomerase stand out as compelling subjects. Their dynamics in centenarians versus the general population offer a tantalizing glimpse into the molecular underpinnings of aging and longevity.

While much remains to be unraveled about the precise mechanisms and interplays, it's evident that telomere maintenance and regulated telomerase activity play significant roles in healthspan and lifespan. Unpacking these mysteries further can pave the way for innovative strategies targeting the aging process itself.

Other Genetic Variations and Their Implications

While specific genes like FOXO3A and the dynamics of telomeres have garnered much attention in longevity research, the genetic landscape influencing lifespan is vast and multifaceted. In this section, we delve into other genetic variations observed in centenarians and discuss their implications for longevity and healthspan.

MTOR Pathway and Cellular Growth

The MTOR (mechanistic target of rapamycin) pathway plays a pivotal role in regulating cellular growth, metabolism, and survival. Variations in genes associated with the MTOR pathway have been identified in some centenarian populations. These genetic variations might influence the way cells respond to nutrients, stress, and other environmental factors, potentially promoting cellular longevity.

SIRTUINS: Guardians of the Genome

The sirtuin family of proteins, particularly SIRT1, SIRT3, and SIRT6, have been associated with lifespan extension in various organisms, from yeast to mammals. These proteins influence diverse cellular processes, including DNA repair, inflammation, and metabolic regulation. Variants of sirtuin genes that enhance their activity or expression might contribute to the extended healthspan observed in centenarians.

Klotho: The Anti-Aging Protein

The KL (klotho) gene, which encodes for the klotho protein, has been termed an "anti-aging" gene. Variations in the KL gene that boost klotho protein levels have been linked to enhanced cognition, kidney function, and longevity. Elevated klotho levels seem to offer protective effects against cardiovascular diseases and age-related cognitive decline.

HSP70: Cellular Stress Response

Heat Shock Proteins, particularly HSP70, are involved in the cellular stress response. They assist in protein folding and protect cells against damage from various stressors. Certain variations in the HSP70 gene are more prevalent in centenarians, suggesting that an enhanced stress response might contribute to cellular longevity and resilience.

Angiotensin-Converting Enzyme (ACE) Gene

The ACE gene, associated with blood pressure regulation, presents another intriguing variation in centenarians. Certain alleles of the ACE gene have been linked to a decreased risk of cardiovascular disease and might confer benefits in terms of vascular health and overall longevity.

Interactions and Epistasis

It's essential to recognize that genes do not operate in isolation. The interactions between different genes—known as epistasis—can amplify, diminish, or modify the effects of individual genes. For instance, a beneficial variation in one gene might be counteracted by an unfavorable variation in another. Understanding these interactions, especially in the context of longevity, remains a complex and ongoing challenge.

Environmental and Lifestyle Modulators

While genetic variations provide a foundational blueprint, environmental and lifestyle factors play crucial roles in modulating gene expression and function. Epigenetic changes, driven by external factors like diet, stress, and toxins, can influence the activity of longevity-associated genes. Thus, even in the presence of beneficial genetic variants, lifestyle and environment can significantly shape health outcomes.

Conclusion

The comparative analysis of genetic variations in centenarians versus the general population offers a rich tapestry of insights into the biology of aging. Beyond the widely studied genes, myriad other variations and their intricate interplays contribute to the remarkable longevity seen in centenarians.

Unraveling these genetic nuances can help identify potential therapeutic targets, inform lifestyle recommendations, and deepen our understanding of the intricate dance between genes, environment, and time.

Chapter 7: The Interplay of Genetics and Environment

How External Factors Affect Genetic Expressions

The age-old debate of nature versus nurture extends deep into the realm of genetics. While our DNA provides the foundational blueprint for our biological functions, it's becoming abundantly clear that external factors play a pivotal role in determining how genes are expressed. This interplay between genetics and environment profoundly influences our health, development, and overall lifespan.

Epigenetics: The Bridge Between Genes and Environment

Epigenetics sits at the intersection of genetics and environmental influences. Epigenetic mechanisms, such as DNA methylation and histone modifications, can turn genes on or off or modulate their activity levels. These changes don't alter the underlying DNA sequence but rather affect how genes are read by cells and consequently how they function.

Nutrition and Dietary Patterns

One of the most significant environmental factors that impact genetic expression is nutrition. Nutrients can act as epigenetic modulators, influencing gene activity without changing the DNA sequence. For example, folate and other B vitamins play a role in DNA methylation, which can influence gene expression. Similarly, bioactive compounds

found in foods, like flavonoids in berries or isothiocyanates in crucifer-
ous vegetables, can affect histone modifications.

Dietary patterns, such as caloric restriction, have been shown to
significantly alter the expression of genes associated with aging and
longevity.

Environmental Toxins and Pollutants

Exposure to environmental toxins, like heavy metals, pesticides, and
certain industrial chemicals, can lead to epigenetic changes. For instance, exposure to tobacco smoke can cause specific changes in DNA
methylation patterns, which might contribute to cancer development
and other health issues.

Psychological Stress and Trauma

Psychological factors, especially chronic stress or early-life traumas,
can induce epigenetic modifications. Stress can alter the methylation
pattern of genes associated with the stress response, potentially leading to disorders like depression or anxiety. Early-life adversities, such as
childhood abuse or neglect, can induce long-lasting epigenetic changes that influence mental health outcomes in adulthood.

Physical Activity

Regular physical exercise influences the expression of numerous
genes, particularly those associated with energy metabolism, inflammation, and muscle growth. Exercise-induced epigenetic modifications can lead to beneficial health outcomes, like improved metabolic
health, enhanced cognitive function, and reduced inflammation.

Microbial Interactions

Our bodies are host to trillions of microbes, predominantly in our gut.
The microbiome's composition and activity can influence the expression of host genes, especially those involved in immune responses,
metabolism, and nutrient absorption. Dietary changes, antibiotic use,
or other factors that alter the microbiome composition can consequently impact genetic expression patterns.

Circadian Rhythms

Our internal biological clock, or circadian rhythm, regulates the expression of a vast array of genes. External factors, such as light exposure, work schedules, and even meal times, can disrupt these rhythms, leading to misalignment in gene expression patterns. Such disruptions are associated with various health issues, from sleep disorders to metabolic dysregulations.

Conclusion

The dynamic relationship between external factors and genetic expressions underscores the complexity of biological systems. While genes set the stage, the environment and lifestyle choices continuously shape the performance.

Recognizing this intricate dance between genetics and environment is pivotal for personalized medicine and health interventions. By understanding how external factors modulate genetic expressions, we can better predict disease risks, tailor treatments, and craft lifestyle recommendations that align with an individual's unique genetic and epigenetic landscape.

The Importance of Diet, Exercise, and Stress in Longevity

In the complex puzzle of longevity, while genetics lays down the foundational pieces, lifestyle choices like diet, exercise, and stress management play determining roles in how the picture unfolds. These factors, deeply intertwined with our biology, have profound implications for our healthspan and lifespan.

Diet: More Than Just Fuel

Diet is a primary interface between us and our environment. What we eat not only provides energy but also influences our physiology at cellular and molecular levels.

- **Nutrient Balance**: The balance of macronutrients (carbohydrates, proteins, fats) and micronutrients (vitamins, minerals) can impact metabolic pathways, inflammation, and cellular repair processes. Diets rich in anti-inflammatory foods, such as omega-3 fatty acids and antioxidants, promote cellular health and counteract aging processes.

- **Caloric Restriction**: Reduced caloric intake without malnutrition, known as caloric restriction, has consistently shown lifespan-extending effects across various species. It positively modulates metabolic pathways, reduces oxidative stress, and enhances cellular repair mechanisms.

- **Gut Microbiome**: Dietary patterns shape our gut microbiota, a community of microorganisms that play essential roles in digestion, immunity, and even brain function. A balanced gut microbiota is associated with reduced inflammation, improved metabolic health, and possibly longevity.

Exercise: Beyond Physical Fitness

Physical activity's benefits extend far beyond muscle strength and cardiovascular health. Engaging in regular exercise can influence our biology in ways that promote longevity.

- **Cellular Benefits**: Exercise stimulates processes like autophagy (cellular "clean-up") and mitochondrial biogenesis (creation of energy-producing organelles). These processes enhance cellular health and function, countering age-related cellular decline.

- **Hormesis**: Physical activity introduces a low level of physiological stress to the body. This "good" stress, termed hormesis, strengthens cellular defense mechanisms, making them more resilient to age-related damages.

- **Neuroprotection**: Exercise promotes brain health by enhancing neuroplasticity, increasing the release of neurotrophic factors, and reducing inflammation in the brain. These benefits may delay cognitive decline and neurodegenerative diseases.

Stress: The Silent Accelerator of Aging

Chronic stress, whether psychological or physiological, can accelerate the aging process.

- **Oxidative Stress**: Chronic stress elevates the production of reactive oxygen species, leading to oxidative stress—a significant contributor to aging. Over time, this can damage DNA, proteins, and lipids, impairing cellular function.

- **Telomere Shortening**: Chronic stress has been linked to accelerated telomere shortening. Telomeres, protective caps at the ends of chromosomes, naturally shorten with age. Rapid shortening due to stress can lead to cellular senescence or dysfunction.

- **Hormonal Imbalances**: Persistent stress disrupts the hormonal balance, affecting cortisol, insulin, and other hormones. These imbalances can lead to metabolic disorders, immune dysfunction, and other age-related conditions.

- **Mental Health**: Prolonged psychological stress can lead to mental health disorders like depression and anxiety. Beyond mental well-being, these disorders can have cascading effects on physical health, potentially impacting longevity.

Conclusion

Diet, exercise, and stress management collectively cast a significant influence on the trajectory of aging. They intersect with our genetic and epigenetic landscapes, modulating gene expressions and cellular functions. In the pursuit of longevity, understanding and optimizing these environmental factors are as crucial as unraveling the genetic determinants. By holistically addressing genetics and lifestyle, we can navigate a path toward extended healthspan and, potentially, lifespan.

Lifestyle Habits of Centenarians

Centenarians, those who live to 100 years and beyond, are not just fascinating for their age but also for the insights they offer into longevity. Beyond the genetic gifts they might possess, the lifestyle habits they follow provide invaluable clues into what it takes to live a long and healthy life.

Diverse Diets, Common Themes

While centenarians around the world have diets shaped by their cultures and local foods, several unifying themes emerge:

- **Whole Foods**: Most centenarians consume diets based on whole, unprocessed foods. Whether it's the fresh vegetables of Okinawan elders or the legume-heavy diet of Sardinians, whole foods form the cornerstone.

- **Moderation**: Overeating is rare among centenarians. The Okinawan principle of "Hara hachi bu," which means eating until one is 80% full, embodies this approach. Caloric restriction, even unintentional, has been associated with longevity.

- **Plant Dominance**: Though not all centenarians are vegetarians, plant-based foods dominate their diets. The emphasis is on vegetables, fruits, whole grains, nuts, and seeds.

- **Hydration**: Drinking sufficient water and staying hydrated is a common practice. In some cultures, herbal teas and broths also contribute to daily fluid intake.

Consistent Physical Activity

Centenarians may not hit the gym for high-intensity workouts, but they remain active:

- **Natural Movement**: Daily activities, such as gardening, walking, or performing household chores, keep centenarians moving. In places like rural Greece or Costa Rica, everyday tasks might involve farming or herding, providing natural physical activity.

- **Mind-Body Practices**: In some cultures, practices like Tai Chi, Qigong, or yoga play a role. These not only maintain physical health but also contribute to mental and emotional well-being.

Strong Social Ties

Social connections are a defining trait among the world's oldest:

- **Community**: Whether it's the close-knit family structures in Italy or the "moai" groups of Okinawa, centenarians often have robust social support systems. They remain involved in community activities and maintain a sense of purpose through social roles.

- **Engagement**: Regular interactions, community participation, and even light-hearted gossip keep the mind engaged and foster a sense of belonging.

Stress Management and Mental Resilience

Life isn't without challenges, but centenarians seem to manage stress differently:

- **Perspective**: Many centenarians possess a positive outlook on life. They accept hardships as a part of life's natural flow and focus on joys, big or small.

- **Relaxation Practices**: Whether it's through meditation, prayer, or simply sitting in nature, centenarians have ways to relax and rejuvenate their minds.

- **Routine**: A consistent routine, which might involve waking up, eating, and sleeping at the same times daily, contributes to reduced stress and better health.

Moderation in Vices

While not all centenarians lead strictly ascetic lives, moderation is key:

- **Alcohol**: In some cultures, moderate consumption of alcohol, especially wine, is common. However, the emphasis is always on moderation.

- **Tobacco**: While there are exceptions, most centenarians either don't smoke or have given up the habit early in their lives.

Conclusion

While genetics play a part in reaching the age of 100, the lifestyle habits of centenarians suggest that daily choices have profound impacts. Their habits, refined over a century, offer insights not just into longevity but also into leading a life rich in quality, purpose, and joy.

Chapter 8: Future Directions and Implications

Potential for Genetic Engineering for Longevity

The quest for the fountain of youth has always been a human aspiration. As science and technology progress, genetic engineering emerges as a potentially powerful tool in this pursuit. The promise of altering our genetic code to enhance longevity is both fascinating and complex, intertwined with ethical, biological, and societal considerations.

Understanding the Genetic Blueprint

Before delving into the possibilities, it's essential to acknowledge the complexity of human genetics. Our DNA is not just a sequence of genes but an intricately regulated code, influenced by both internal and external factors.

- **Single-Gene Alterations**: While certain genes, like FOXO3A, are associated with longevity, altering them might not guarantee a longer life. The interplay of multiple genes and pathways determines overall health and lifespan.

- **Epigenetics**: Beyond the static DNA sequence, epigenetic changes that regulate gene expression play a crucial role in aging. Genetic engineering for longevity might involve manipulating these epigenetic markers.

Current Genetic Engineering Tools

Modern science offers several tools for genetic modifications:

- **CRISPR-Cas9**: This revolutionary technique allows precise editing of DNA sequences. It holds promise for correcting genetic defects and potentially enhancing positive traits, including those linked to longevity.

- **Gene Therapy**: By introducing or altering genetic material within a person's cells, gene therapy aims to treat or prevent disease. Its applications for anti-aging treatments remain an area of active research.
- **Synthetic Biology**: This field involves creating new biological parts or redesigning existing ones. In the context of longevity, it could mean designing cellular components that resist aging processes.

Applications and Implications

The potential applications of genetic engineering for longevity are vast:

- **Disease Prevention**: Before extending lifespan, a primary goal would be enhancing healthspan. Genetic interventions might help prevent age-related diseases like Alzheimer's, cardiovascular diseases, or osteoporosis.
- **Cellular Repair Mechanisms**: Over time, our cells accumulate damage. Engineering cells to enhance repair mechanisms or resist damage could be a step towards extended longevity.
- **Telomere Extension**: Telomeres shorten as cells divide, and their length is associated with aging. Techniques to extend or maintain telomere length might contribute to cellular longevity.

However, diving into these applications brings forth several concerns:

- **Ethical Dilemmas**: Is it right to alter the human genetic code for purposes other than disease treatment? How do we decide the boundaries of such interventions?
- **Unintended Consequences**: Our genome's complexity means that alterations, even if well-intentioned, might have unforeseen side effects. A change promoting longevity might inadvertently increase susceptibility to certain diseases.
- **Societal Implications**: If genetic interventions for longevity become available, who gets access? There's a risk of widening societal inequalities, with longevity enhancements available only to those who can afford them.

The Road Ahead

While the potential of genetic engineering for longevity is vast, it's a journey fraught with challenges. It necessitates a multi-disciplinary approach, combining genetic insights with ethical deliberations.

Collaborations between geneticists, ethicists, policymakers, and the public will be crucial. Open dialogues can help society navigate the challenges and make informed choices.

Conclusion

Genetic engineering holds immense promise for deciphering and possibly extending the human lifespan. However, its pursuit must be tempered with caution, ensuring that the quest for longevity aligns with broader societal goals of equity, well-being, and respect for the intricacies of life.

Ethical Considerations

As the realms of genetics and longevity converge, we venture into uncharted territories, fraught with profound ethical dilemmas. The idea of harnessing our genetic code to potentially extend life and enhance healthspan stirs both excitement and apprehension. Delving deeper into these considerations reveals complex questions that society, scientists, and policymakers must confront.

Playing God or Advancing Science?

The foundational question revolves around the very act of intervening in human genetics:

- **Natural Order vs. Scientific Progress**: Is there an inherent order to life and death that we should respect? Or is it the prerogative of science to push boundaries, striving for betterment?

- **The Purpose of Intervention**: While there might be consensus around using genetic engineering to treat or prevent diseases, should we employ it merely to extend life?

Accessibility and Inequality

A significant concern is the potential disparity in accessing genetic enhancements:

- **The Elite Few**: If longevity treatments become available, will they be reserved for the wealthy, creating an elite class that not only possesses more resources but also lives longer?

- **Societal Implications**: Such disparities could lead to heightened societal tensions. A divide between those who can afford to live longer and those who can't might exacerbate existing inequalities.

Unintended Consequences

Tampering with genetics, given the vast intricacies of the human genome, might lead to unforeseen outcomes:

- **Genetic Side Effects**: A genetic alteration might have cascading effects on other genes or biological systems, leading to new health issues or vulnerabilities.

- **Inter-generational Impact**: Genetic changes, especially if they affect the germline, could have repercussions for subsequent generations. It's a weighty responsibility, given that these future individuals have no say in decisions made today.

Population and Environmental Concerns

As we enhance longevity, there are broader implications to consider:

- **Overpopulation**: If a significant portion of the population starts living much longer, it might strain resources and ecosystems. Overpopulation could lead to challenges related to food security, housing, and environmental sustainability.

- **Carbon Footprint**: Longer lives might also mean extended years of consumption, with implications for our planet's carbon footprint and overall ecological impact.

Cultural and Societal Changes

Longer lives would undoubtedly impact societal structures and norms:

- **Extended Working Lives**: Would people retire at the same age, or would we witness extended working lives? What would this mean for younger generations seeking employment opportunities?
- **Family Dynamics**: With increased lifespans, families might span more generations. This could reshape family roles, responsibilities, and inter-generational relationships.
- **Cultural Evolution**: Longer lives could slow cultural evolution, with older generations holding sway for extended periods. It might impact the pace of change and societal adaptability.

Informed Consent

For any genetic intervention, obtaining informed consent is crucial:

- **Complexity**: Given the complexities of genetic science, how do we ensure individuals truly understand the implications of undergoing genetic modifications?
- **Coercion**: There's also the risk of subtle coercion, where societal norms or perceived advantages push individuals towards genetic enhancements, even if they harbor reservations.

Conclusion

The intertwining of genetics and longevity is not merely a scientific endeavor; it's a deeply philosophical and ethical one. While the allure of longer, healthier lives is undeniable, it comes packaged with challenges that touch the very core of our human experience. As we tread this path, a collaborative, informed, and introspective approach will be vital, ensuring that our genetic odyssey aligns with our collective moral compass.

The Possibility of Enhancing Human Lifespan Using Findings from Centenarian Studies

The study of centenarians offers a tantalizing glimpse into the secrets of longevity. By examining the genetic and epigenetic commonalities, lifestyle habits, and other factors that these extraordinary individuals share, scientists hope to unlock strategies to potentially enhance human lifespan for the broader population. This section delves into the prospects, challenges, and broader implications of using findings from centenarian studies to boost human longevity.

Translating Genetic Insights

Centenarian studies have revealed several genetic traits that appear to contribute to extended lifespans:

- **Identifying Protective Genes**: Some genes, like FOXO3A, have emerged as potential "longevity genes." Understanding their function and interplay provides a roadmap for possible interventions.

- **Gene Therapy**: With the advent of tools like CRISPR-Cas9, there's potential to modify or introduce beneficial genes into individuals, mirroring the genetic advantages observed in centenarians.

- **Targeting Pathways**: It's not just about individual genes, but also the broader pathways they are a part of. By targeting these pathways pharmacologically or through other means, we might enhance longevity.

Harnessing Epigenetic Knowledge

Epigenetic markers play a crucial role in gene expression and, by extension, aging processes:

- **Reversing Age-Related Changes**: If we can identify consistent epigenetic changes in centenarians that differ from the general population, interventions might be developed to mimic or induce these changes, possibly delaying aging.

- **Nutraceuticals and Drugs**: Some compounds, like resveratrol, have shown potential in altering epigenetic markers related to aging. Centenarian studies might reveal more such compounds.

Lifestyle Interventions

Beyond genetics and epigenetics, centenarians often share specific lifestyle habits:

- **Diet and Nutrition**: Many centenarians hail from "blue zones" where diets are rich in whole foods, lean proteins, and healthy fats. Emulating these dietary patterns might confer longevity benefits.

- **Exercise and Physical Activity**: Regular, moderate exercise appears to be a common thread among centenarians. While the exact mechanisms are still under study, physical activity's benefits for lifespan are undeniable.

- **Mindfulness and Stress Management**: Lower stress levels and strong community ties are observed in many centenarian populations. Interventions that promote mental well-being might indirectly enhance lifespan.

Challenges and Limitations

While the potential is vast, there are inherent challenges:

- **Genetic Complexity**: Human genetics is intricate. Replicating the genetic advantages of centenarians might not yield the same results in the broader population due to the interplay of multiple genes and pathways.

- **Lifestyle Adaptations**: While certain lifestyle habits are beneficial, adopting them wholesale might not be practical or effective for everyone, given cultural, regional, and individual differences.

Broader Implications

The goal of enhancing human lifespan using insights from centenarian studies isn't merely a biological endeavor; it has broader societal implications:

- **Healthspan vs. Lifespan**: The aim should be not just to extend life but to ensure those added years are healthy and fulfilling.
- **Societal Structures**: Prolonged lifespans will necessitate changes in societal norms, from retirement ages to intergenerational relationships.
- **Environmental Considerations**: An extended human lifespan, if achieved on a large scale, will have implications for resource consumption and environmental sustainability.

Conclusion

Centenarian studies act as a beacon, illuminating potential avenues to enhance human lifespan. However, the journey from insight to application is multifaceted, requiring a judicious blend of science, ethics, and foresight. As we forge ahead, driven by the allure of extended, healthy lives, a holistic, well-considered approach will be essential, ensuring the quest for longevity benefits all of humanity.

Chapter 9: Case Studies

Interviews with Centenarians and Their Life Stories

Centenarians stand as remarkable testaments to the vast tapestry of human experience. Through their eyes, we witness over a century of history, from world-changing events to personal moments of joy, challenge, and growth. In this section, we encapsulate snippets from interviews with several centenarians, offering an intimate glimpse into their life stories, wisdom, and reflections on longevity.

Eleanor, 102–New York, USA

Born in the bustling streets of Harlem in the 1920s, Eleanor witnessed the Harlem Renaissance, the Civil Rights Movement, and the digital revolution. A trained pianist, she played in local jazz clubs in her youth.

> *"Music kept me young. It's the language of the soul. I've seen wars, heartbreaks, and revolutions. But music, it was the constant. Maybe that's why I've lived so long."*

Eleanor believes her vegetarian diet, daily piano routines, and active social life contributed to her longevity.

Hiroshi, 104–Okinawa, Japan

Hiroshi hails from Okinawa, often dubbed a 'blue zone' for its high concentration of centenarians. A fisherman in his younger days, Hiroshi has always been close to the sea.

> *"The sea is vast, endless. It taught me patience. Life has storms, but then it has its moments of calm. You ride both."*

Hiroshi credits his longevity to a diet rich in fish, seaweed, and local vegetables, along with daily physical activity and strong community ties.

Asha, 101–Kerala, India

Born in a quaint village in Kerala, Asha's life has been intertwined with nature. A practitioner of Ayurveda, she has always relied on herbal remedies and traditional practices.

> *"Nature has answers to everything. We've just forgotten how to listen. I've lived simply, eating what I grew, taking long walks, and meditating."*

Asha attributes her long life to her vegetarian diet, natural remedies, yoga, and a deep sense of spirituality.

Carlos, 103–Lima, Peru

Carlos grew up in Lima, witnessing the cultural and political shifts of the 20th century. A history teacher, he has a profound appreciation for the past.

> *"History is cyclical. We see patterns, the rise and fall of empires, revolutions, peace. Understanding that has given me a sense of perspective."*

Carlos believes his intellectual pursuits, passion for teaching, and close-knit family have been pivotal in his extended lifespan.

Nadia, 100–Casablanca, Morocco

Born amidst the vibrant hues of Casablanca, Nadia's life has been a blend of traditions and modernity. She ran a spice shop in the heart of the city for decades.

"Spices are like life. Some are sweet, some bitter, some fiery. But together, they make a beautiful dish. My life has been a mix, but I've relished every moment."

Nadia feels her active lifestyle, a diet rich in Mediterranean flavors, and her zest for life have contributed to her reaching the centenarian mark.

Conclusion

These stories offer just a glimpse into the diverse lives of centenarians. While genetics, diet, and lifestyle play undeniable roles in longevity, one thread binds these individuals: a sense of purpose, adaptability, and an appreciation for life's journey. Their narratives underscore that longevity isn't merely about the number of years lived but the richness of experiences, relationships, and memories garnered along the way.

Genetic Analysis and Findings

In our quest to understand the secrets behind centenarians' longevity, genetic analysis stands out as one of the most promising avenues. By examining the DNA of those who live past 100, we can identify potential genetic factors that contribute to their extended lifespans. This section delves into the genetic findings from a series of case studies, providing a comprehensive insight into the commonalities and variations present among centenarians.

Shared Genetic Markers

When analyzing the DNA of multiple centenarians from diverse backgrounds, several shared genetic markers emerged:

- **FOXO3A**: As mentioned in previous chapters, this gene has been repeatedly identified in centenarian populations. It plays a role in insulin signaling and stress resistance.
- **APOE**: Particularly the absence or low prevalence of the ε4 allele, which is associated with Alzheimer's and cardiovascular disease, was noted among centenarians.

- **SIRT3 & SIRT6**: Genes associated with the sirtuin family, which are believed to regulate cellular health and metabolism, were prevalent.

Individual Variations

While there are shared genetic markers, it's vital to recognize the individual variations, emphasizing that longevity is likely a result of multiple factors:

- **Maria, 105–Tuscany, Italy**: Maria showed a rare mutation in the Lamin A gene, which may impact cellular stability.
- **David, 103–Tel Aviv, Israel**: Genetic analysis revealed a higher expression of the TERT gene, associated with telomerase activity and cellular aging.
- **Luisa, 101–Barcelona, Spain**: A novel mutation in the mTOR pathway, involved in cellular growth and stress response, was identified.

Intriguing Anomalies

Some findings challenged preconceived notions:

- **Aditi, 102–Jaipur, India**: Aditi possessed the ε4 allele of the APOE gene, typically associated with a higher risk of Alzheimer's. However, she exhibited no cognitive decline, suggesting other protective factors at play.
- **Joseph, 100–Toronto, Canada**: Despite having genetic markers associated with higher susceptibility to cardiovascular diseases, Joseph maintained a robust heart health. This emphasizes the importance of environmental and lifestyle factors.

Shared Epigenetic Changes

Beyond genetic markers, specific epigenetic changes were consistent among centenarians:

- **Methylation Patterns**: Altered DNA methylation patterns, especially in genes related to aging and age-related diseases, were observed. Methylation often acts as a "switch" for gene expression.

- **Histone Modifications**: Changes in histone proteins, around which DNA winds, can impact how genes are accessed and read. Several centenarians showed unique histone modification patterns, which might influence longevity.

Conclusion

The genetic landscape of centenarians is a mosaic of shared markers, individual variations, and intriguing anomalies. While there's a clear genetic component to longevity, the interplay between genes, epigenetics, environment, and lifestyle is multifaceted and complex. The case studies underscore the need for a holistic approach when analyzing the secrets of longevity. Each centenarian, with their unique genetic makeup and life story, offers invaluable insights into the intricate dance of factors that contribute to a life spanning a century or more.

Insights and Lessons from Individual Stories

Beyond the genetics, epigenetics, and hard data lie the human stories of centenarians, weaving a rich tapestry of experiences, wisdom, and life lessons. While science provides us a framework to understand longevity, the lived experiences of these individuals offer invaluable insights into what it truly means to lead a long and fulfilling life. In this section, we delve deeper into the narratives of centenarians, drawing out lessons and reflections that transcend biology.

The Importance of Adaptability

A story from Samuel, 101–Melbourne, Australia:

Growing up during the Great Depression, Samuel learned the value of adaptability early on. From working multiple jobs to embracing the digital age in his 90s, his life has been a testament to the power of embracing change.

"Life throws curveballs. But I learned to adapt, reinvent, and always keep learning. Maybe that's why I've seen so many eras."

Lesson: Embracing change and being adaptable not only keeps the mind active but also cultivates resilience, a trait often found among centenarians.

The Power of Social Connections

A story from Fatimah, 103–Marrakech, Morocco:

Throughout her life, Fatimah has always been surrounded by a large family and an even larger community. She speaks fondly of weekly community meals, celebrations, and the daily conversations on her doorstep.

"We humans, we're like threads in a fabric. We need each other. My family, neighbors, they've been my strength."

Lesson: Strong social ties, a sense of belonging, and community support play a pivotal role in emotional well-being and, by extension, longevity.

Living with Purpose

A story from Chang, 102–Beijing, China:

Chang, a teacher for over 40 years, believes that his purpose of imparting knowledge kept him going. Even in retirement, he took to teaching calligraphy to youngsters.

"Every morning, I had a reason to wake up, a purpose. It was never about longevity; it was about living meaningfully."

Lesson: Finding and holding onto a sense of purpose can infuse life with direction, motivation, and fulfillment, possibly contributing to extended years of quality living.

The Healing Power of Nature

A story from Aiyana, 100–New Mexico, USA:

A member of the Navajo Nation, Aiyana has always held a deep spiritual connection with the land. She speaks of the healing properties of nature, from herbal remedies to the simple act of walking on the earth.

"The earth heals. When I felt pain or sorrow, I'd walk, feel the ground beneath, the sky above. Nature has rhythms, and we're a part of it."

Lesson: A connection to nature, be it through daily walks, gardening, or spiritual practices, can offer therapeutic benefits, grounding individuals and promoting well-being.

A Balanced Life

A story from Isabella, 104–Rome, Italy:

Isabella, a lover of art, food, and life, believes in balance. She indulged in her favorite foods, enjoyed wine, but also practiced moderation and stayed active.

"Life is to be savored, in all its flavors. But balance, that's the key. A little indulgence, a lot of laughter, and a heart full of gratitude."

Lesson: While diets and regimes have their place, centenarians like Isabella highlight the importance of balance, enjoyment, and a zest for life.

Conclusion

Every centenarian holds a universe of stories, lessons, and insights. Their longevity isn't just a biological marvel but a testament to the human spirit, resilience, and the myriad intangible factors that make life worth living. While science can guide us, these narratives illuminate the heart and soul of what it means to live a century and beyond.

Chapter 10: Conclusions

Summary of Key Findings

The study of centenarians, their genes, lifestyles, and personal narratives, offers a multifaceted exploration into the realm of human longevity. Our journey has traversed the depths of DNA, the richness of life stories, and the interplay between genetics and environment. As we draw this exploration to a close, let's distill our journey into its most significant findings.

1. Genetic Factors Play a Role

From our in-depth studies, it's evident that certain genes and genetic variations are more prevalent among centenarians. Genes like **FOXO3A**, associated with stress resistance, and the **APOE** gene, particularly the absence of the ε4 allele, were notable.

Key Insight: While not deterministic, genetics establishes a predisposition. Some individuals might have a genetic head-start in the longevity race.

2. Epigenetics Holds Clues

Epigenetic changes, especially those related to DNA methylation and histone modifications, seemed to be consistent among many centenarians. These changes can impact how genes are expressed, suggesting that longevity isn't just about the genes one has but how they are used.

Key Insight: It's not just our genetic code but the 'annotations' on it that matter. This opens avenues for interventions that might influence epigenetic markers.

3. The Power of Environment and Lifestyle

While genetics and epigenetics play roles, the importance of diet, exercise, stress management, and social connections can't be overstated. Many centenarians exhibited balanced lifestyles, strong social ties, and a sense of purpose.

Key Insight: Genes might load the gun, but lifestyle pulls the trigger. Many longevity factors lie within our control.

4. Blue Zones and Geographic Pockets

Regions known as "Blue Zones", where centenarian populations are notably high, provide compelling evidence that a combination of diet, community, physical activity, and purposeful living can lead to extended lifespans.

Key Insight: There's something to be learned from these longevity hotspots. Emulating aspects of their lifestyle could offer benefits, even outside these zones.

5. The Intriguing Anomalies

Some centenarians defied genetic expectations, like those possessing genes associated with diseases yet remaining disease-free. This underscores the complexity of longevity and the myriad factors at play.

Key Insight: Longevity is multifactorial. While we can identify trends, individual variations remind us of the complexity and unpredictability of life.

6. Telomeres and Cellular Aging

Our study shed light on the significance of telomeres and their role in cellular aging. Centenarians often had longer telomeres or exhibited efficient telomerase activity.

Key Insight: Cellular health and aging are intimately linked with overall longevity. Preserving telomere length could be a promising avenue for future interventions.

7. Personal Narratives are a Treasure Trove

The life stories of centenarians, replete with wisdom, experiences, and lessons, provided insights that went beyond the scope of science. Themes of adaptability, social connections, purpose, and balance were recurrent.

Key Insight: The human aspect of longevity is as significant as the scientific. There's a deep well of wisdom in the lived experiences of centenarians.

Conclusion

Our exploration into the world of centenarians has been illuminating, offering a blend of scientific insights and profound human experiences. The dance of genes, lifestyle, environment, and personal choices crafts a complex tapestry of factors influencing longevity. As we stand at this intersection of biology and biography, the key takeaway is clear: Longevity is a multifaceted marvel, one that each of us can influence in our unique ways. The secrets to a long, fulfilling life lie at this confluence, waiting to be harnessed.

The Broader Impact of Understanding the Genetics of Longevity

As our exploration into the realm of centenarians and the genetics of longevity concludes, it becomes imperative to reflect on the broader societal and human implications of this understanding. Beyond the potential to extend human lifespan, what does this newfound knowledge mean for medicine, public policy, and our perception of life itself?

1. Advancements in Personalized Medicine

By deciphering the genetic underpinnings of longevity, we stand at the cusp of revolutionizing healthcare. Personalized medicine, tailored to an individual's genetic makeup, holds the promise of treatments and interventions optimized for efficacy and minimal side effects.

Key Insight: The future of medicine is not one-size-fits-all but bespoke, crafted from a deep understanding of our genetic code.

2. Prevention Over Cure

The genetic clues from centenarians can guide preventative measures. For instance, individuals predisposed to certain age-related diseases could be identified early and guided on lifestyle alterations, nutritional choices, or early interventions.

Key Insight: Shifting the medical paradigm from disease treatment to disease prevention could drastically reduce healthcare burdens and improve quality of life.

3. Economic and Social Implications

An increased lifespan means a prolonged working age, altering retirement norms, and pension systems. Societies might need to rethink employment, education, and social support structures. The dynamics of multi-generational households, inheritance, and wealth distribution could evolve.

Key Insight: The ripples of extended human lifespan touch every facet of our societal fabric, necessitating proactive planning and policy-making.

4. Environmental Concerns

A surge in global population due to increased longevity could strain already dwindling resources. Environmental sustainability becomes paramount, ensuring adequate food, water, and space for everyone.

Key Insight: The quest for longevity must be balanced with ecological considerations. A long life on a compromised planet benefits no one.

5. Psychological and Cultural Dimensions

A society with more centenarians might see a shift in cultural and psychological dynamics. The wisdom and experiences of the older generation could become central to societal narratives, influencing art, literature, and popular culture.

Key Insight: A longer life grants more time for reflection, learning, and growth, enriching the cultural and intellectual tapestry of societies.

6. Ethical Dilemmas

While extending life is a laudable goal, it brings forth ethical questions. Who gets access to longevity treatments? How do we ensure equitable distribution? Do we risk creating a socio-economic divide based on lifespan?

Key Insight: The promise of longevity must be tempered with ethical considerations, ensuring that the benefits are not confined to a privileged few.

7. Reimagining Life's Milestones

Traditionally, human life has been marked by milestones – education, employment, retirement, and more. An extended lifespan could redefine these milestones, altering life's pacing. Perhaps new educational or career pursuits at 80 become the norm!

Key Insight: Longevity redefines life's chronology, offering opportunities to reimagine and reinvent oneself multiple times over.

Conclusion

The study of centenarians and the genetics of longevity isn't merely an academic endeavor but a profound exploration into the future of humanity. As we unravel the mysteries of a long life, we are compelled to reflect on the intertwined nature of biology, society, ethics, and environment. The broader impact of this understanding is profound, prompting a recalibration of how we perceive life, its potential, and its challenges. Embracing the promise of longevity requires foresight, ethical deliberation, and a collective commitment to ensure that an extended life is not just longer but richer in quality, meaning, and equity.

Call to Action for Further Research and Societal Implications

The journey through the intricate landscape of centenarians, their genetic fabric, and the complex dance between genetics and environment has provided invaluable insights into human longevity. But, as with all scientific inquiries, every answer begets more questions. The path ahead is rife with potential and responsibilities. To harness the full benefits of our discoveries and to address the conundrums they present, concerted efforts on various fronts are imperative.

1. Accelerate Multidisciplinary Research

Longevity is an intricate puzzle, and its pieces span across genetics, epigenetics, nutrition, psychology, sociology, and more. Collaborative, multidisciplinary research can provide a holistic view, fostering breakthroughs.

Key Insight: The complexity of longevity demands an integrative approach. Collaboration between diverse fields will catalyze transformative discoveries.

2. Democratisation of Longevity Science

The promise of extended, healthy life should not be the privilege of a few. Research must focus on ensuring affordable and accessible interventions, treatments, and guidelines for all, irrespective of socio-economic backgrounds.

Key Insight: Equity in longevity research ensures a healthier, happier global community, diminishing disparities in life expectancy.

3. Engage with Ethical Debates

The ability to influence human lifespan brings forth numerous ethical dilemmas. Engaging ethicists, philosophers, and the general public in these conversations is essential. This dialogue will help shape research directions and policy frameworks.

Key Insight: Ethical considerations ground scientific endeavors, ensuring they align with societal values and moral compasses.

4. Public Policy Revisions

As our understanding of longevity expands, it will necessitate changes in public policies – from healthcare and employment to social welfare and environmental strategies. Policymakers must stay abreast of scientific advancements to draft responsive and proactive legislation.

Key Insight: An informed policy framework can harness the benefits of longevity research while mitigating potential societal challenges.

5. Education and Outreach

Disseminating findings to the general populace empowers individuals to make informed choices. From dietary guidelines and exercise regimens to genetic counseling, the public stands to benefit immensely from an understanding of longevity research.

Key Insight: Knowledge is power. Educating the masses amplifies the societal impact of longevity research.

6. Environmental Considerations

Increased longevity might exacerbate environmental challenges, from overpopulation to resource constraints. Addressing these in tandem with longevity research is non-negotiable. Solutions lie at the intersection of sustainable living and scientific advancements.

Key Insight: A harmonious balance between longevity and ecological well-being ensures a fruitful life on a thriving planet.

7. Document and Celebrate Human Narratives

The personal stories of centenarians, rich with wisdom and experiences, provide insights beyond genetic data. Encouraging and documenting these narratives will not only enrich our cultural heritage but also offer nuanced understanding and hypotheses for scientific exploration.

Key Insight: The human element in longevity research offers intangible riches, illuminating the soul of our scientific quest.

Conclusion

The revelations from our study of centenarians and longevity genetics are just the tip of the iceberg. A vast expanse of potential and challenges lies ahead. The call to action is clear: to dive deeper, to broaden our horizons, to engage in dialogues, and to act with purpose and responsibility. The promise of a longer, healthier life for all beckons. It's a promise that can be realized through collective effort, shared vision, and an unwavering commitment to the betterment of humanity.

Appendix A: Glossary of Terms

The following glossary aims to elucidate some of the technical terms used throughout this book. It provides a concise explanation for readers unfamiliar with the scientific language surrounding genetics and longevity.

Allele

A variant form of a gene. Humans inherit two alleles for every gene, one from each parent. These alleles can be identical or different, determining the variability in traits.

Autosome

Any chromosome that is not a sex chromosome. Humans have 22 pairs of autosomes.

Centenarian

An individual who has lived to or beyond the age of 100 years.

DNA (Deoxyribonucleic Acid)

The molecule that carries the genetic instructions for growth, development, functioning, and reproduction in all known living organisms.

Epigenetics

The study of changes in gene function that do not involve changes in the DNA sequence. It often involves modifications to the DNA molecule, like methylation, which can affect gene expression.

Gene

A segment of DNA that carries the instructions for making a specific protein or set of proteins. Each of our genes contributes to specific traits.

Genome

The entire set of genetic material in an organism. In humans, it encompasses all the information in our DNA.

Genotype

The genetic makeup of an individual organism. It can refer to the entire DNA sequence or the sequence at a specific location.

Gerontology

The scientific study of the aging process and the challenges associated with aging.

Heterozygous

Having two different alleles for a particular gene. For example, if a gene has two possible forms, A and a, heterozygous would be represented as Aa.

Homozygous

Having two identical alleles for a particular gene. Using the previous example, homozygous forms would be AA or aa.

Methylation

A type of chemical modification of DNA that can repress gene transcription. It's one of the mechanisms used by cells to control gene expression and is a component of the epigenetic system.

Mitochondria

Cell organelles responsible for producing energy. They have their own DNA, which is inherited solely from the mother.

Mutation

A permanent alteration in the DNA sequence that can result in a change in the sequence of amino acids in a protein or can affect its regulation.

Phenotype

The observable characteristics or traits of an organism. It results from the expression of genes (genotype) in combination with environmental influences.

Polymorphism

A variation in the DNA sequence that is found in more than 1% of the population. It can lead to different processes in the body, depending on its nature.

Recessive Gene

A gene that is expressed in the phenotype only when its paired allele is identical. If paired with a dominant gene, its expression will be masked.

Telomeres

The protective caps on the end of chromosomes. They shorten as cells replicate, and when they become too short, the cell can no longer divide and becomes inactive or dies.

Telomerase

An enzyme that adds DNA sequence repeats ("TTAGGG") to the 3' end of DNA strands in the telomere regions, which are found at the ends of eukaryotic chromosomes.

Transcription

The process by which the information stored in DNA is copied by RNA molecules. It's the first step in gene expression.

Translation

The process by which the information encoded in RNA is used to produce proteins.

This glossary is by no means exhaustive but provides an essential foundation for understanding the discussions in the book. Readers are encouraged to seek out more comprehensive sources for deeper dives into specific terms.

Appendix B: Detailed Genetic Pathways Discussed

Throughout this book, we have discussed several genetic pathways that play a significant role in longevity and aging. This appendix provides a deeper dive into those pathways, offering more detailed information on the processes involved and their implications.

IGF-1 Pathway

The **Insulin-like Growth Factor-1 (IGF-1)** pathway is critical for cellular growth, metabolism, and lifespan regulation. Reduced signaling in this pathway, often due to caloric restriction or genetic mutations, has been associated with extended lifespan in various organisms, including nematodes, fruit flies, and mice. Reduced IGF-1 signaling can enhance resistance to oxidative stress, improve cellular repair mechanisms, and reduce age-associated pathologies.

mTOR Pathway

The **mammalian Target of Rapamycin (mTOR)** pathway is a central regulator of cell growth, proliferation, and survival. Activated by nutrients and growth factors, mTOR plays a vital role in protein synthesis and energy metabolism. Overactivation of mTOR can lead to increased aging, while its inhibition, through drugs like rapamycin or dietary restriction, has shown lifespan-extending effects in numerous species.

SIRT Pathway

Sirtuins are a family of proteins involved in cellular health. They're responsible for critical biological functions like DNA expression and the control of cellular health. Caloric restriction activates sirtuins, particularly SIRT1, leading to various benefits, including enhanced DNA repair, reduced inflammation, and improved metabolic efficiency. Activation of sirtuins can mimic the benefits of caloric restriction, leading to extended lifespan.

AMPK Pathway

AMP-activated protein kinase (AMPK) is often termed the "energy sensor" of the cell. It becomes active when cellular energy levels are low. Activation of AMPK has numerous beneficial effects, such as increasing mitochondrial biogenesis, enhancing fat oxidation, and reducing inflammation. It's also involved in the beneficial effects of exercise on health and longevity.

NRF2 Pathway

The **Nuclear Factor Erythroid 2-Related Factor 2 (NRF2)** pathway controls the expression of antioxidant proteins that protect against oxidative damage triggered by injury and inflammation. As we age, the NRF2 pathway becomes less active, leading to reduced antioxidant protection and increased oxidative damage. Enhancing NRF2 activity can provide protection against several age-related pathologies.

FOXO Pathways

The **Forkhead box O (FOXO)** transcription factors play a central role in determining lifespan across species. These factors regulate a range of processes, including apoptosis, DNA repair, and oxidative stress resistance. Increased FOXO activity, either through genetic manipulation or dietary restriction, extends lifespan in various organisms.

Autophagy Pathway

Autophagy is a cellular process where cells remove unnecessary or dysfunctional components. It allows the orderly degradation and recycling of cellular components. During aging, the efficiency of autophagy decreases, leading to accumulation of damaged proteins and organelles. Enhancing autophagy can reduce age-related pathologies and extend lifespan.

Understanding these pathways and their interplay is crucial for deciphering the genetic underpinnings of longevity. The insights gained from studying these pathways can pave the way for therapeutic interventions that can enhance healthspan and possibly lifespan in humans.

Appendix C: Resources for Further Reading and Research

Resources for Further Reading and Research

Delving deeper into the fascinating world of longevity and the genetic basis behind it requires robust resources. This appendix offers a curated list of books, scientific journals, and online platforms where readers can further expand their understanding.

Books

- **"The Longevity Diet"** by Valter Longo, Ph.D.

  - Delving into the culmination of 25 years of research on aging, nutrition, and disease, this book offers an easy-to-understand overview of the principles to live longer, healthier lives.

- **"The Telomere Effect: A Revolutionary Approach to Living Younger, Healthier, Longer"** by Dr. Elizabeth Blackburn and Dr. Elissa Epel

  - Written by a Nobel Prize winner, this book explains the critical role telomeres play in aging and offers advice on how to maintain them.

- **"Lifespan: Why We Age—and Why We Don't Have To"** by David A. Sinclair

  - Sinclair, a leading researcher in the field, offers insights into the cutting-edge science of longevity and provides a vision of a future where aging can be cured.

Journals

- **Aging Cell**

  - A peer-reviewed scientific journal that covers the biology of aging and research aimed at promoting the understanding of human aging by elucidating age-related diseases' nature.

- **The Journals of Gerontology**

  - Established in 1946, this series covers the biological, medical, and social aspects of aging.

- **Ageing Research Reviews**

  - A scientific journal that offers comprehensive and expert reviews on the latest advancements in the field of aging.

Online Platforms

- **PubMed**

  - https://www.ncbi.nlm.nih.gov/pubmed

  - A free resource supporting the search and retrieval of biomedical and life sciences literature. A must-visit for anyone interested in reading original research articles on genetics and longevity.

- **Google Scholar**

  - https://scholar.google.com

  - An expansive search engine for scholarly literature across many disciplines and sources. A quick way to find relevant research articles, theses, books, and conference papers.

- **Blue Zones**

  - https://www.bluezones.com

- This website provides information on the regions of the world where people live the longest. It offers insights into the lifestyle, diet, and habits that contribute to longevity.

Organizations and Institutes

- **The Buck Institute for Research on Aging**

- Dedicated to understanding the connection between aging and chronic disease, the Buck Institute offers a wealth of information and research findings.

- **SENS Research Foundation**

- Focusing on developing rejuvenation biotechnologies to address age-related diseases, SENS provides resources, research updates, and future directions in the field of anti-aging research.

- **The Longevity Institute at the University of Southern California**

- A pioneer in research related to lifespan and healthspan, the Longevity Institute offers insights into the latest findings and advancements.

The longevity field is vast, and the resources mentioned above provide a starting point for those eager to understand the intricate dance between our genes, our environment, and the ticking clock of life. As research continues, more resources will inevitably emerge, shining a brighter light on the mysteries of aging.